Slaughter of the Innocents

Child Abuse through the Ages and Today

Slaughter of the Innocents

Child Abuse through the Ages and Today

Sander J. Breiner, M.D.

Plenum Press • New York and London

Library of Congress Cataloging in Publication Data

Breiner, Sander J.
    Slaughter of the innocents: child abuse through the ages and today / Sander J.
Breiner.
        p.   cm.
    Includes bibliographical references.
    ISBN 0-306-43459-8
    1. Child abuse—History—Cross-cultural studies. 2. Social history—To 500. I.
Title.
HV6626.5.B74   1990   89-29451
362.7′6′09—dc20   CIP

© 1990 Sander J. Breiner
Plenum Press is a Division of
Plenum Publishing Corporation
233 Spring Street, New York, N.Y. 10013

Printed in the United States of America

TO MY GRANDCHILDREN

Preface

This book has been dedicated to my grandchildren, and, in truth, to all the grandchildren in the world, including those yet to be born. What is contained herein had to be written. It is only by our understanding of what has taken place in the past and in the present day that we may be able to better protect and nurture all these children. These better-nurtured children, when they mature, are more likely to produce a healthier world for all my grandchildren.

Benjamin Disraeli, the famous Victorian British Prime Minister, said, "What we learn from history, is that we don't learn from history." This must be proved untrue if we wish to advance to a less hurtful phase of civilization.

While the literature related to each of the five civilizations we will examine is already vast, this book makes an unusual contribution in at least three ways. First, it considers all five civilizations in a single volume, facilitating comparisons. Second, it focuses specifically on the seldom-discussed practices of infanticide and child abuse, drawing together references that have been scattered in scores of studies.

Finally, in my interpretation of the historical evidence and the vast secondary literature, I have been able to draw on my training and nearly 30 years of practice as a psychiatrist. Thus the historical approach is augmented by knowledge from contemporary psychiatric theory and practice. Given the rudimentary state of psychohistorical interpretation of the ancient world, I believe this approach may offer significant new insights into the practices of our ancestors.

The following pages will, it is hoped, be interesting, contain information new to you, and providentially help you to see how we all can make important changes in the world of our grandchildren.

Acknowledgments

I didn't start to write a book. It all began with an interest in China. With my studies of that culture and trips to mainland China (1979) and to Hong Kong, Macao, and Taiwan (1974), along with my years of interest in and study of children (their development and problems), I presented psychological studies of these topics to my colleagues.

Each presentation and publication elicited informed and interested response which added to my knowledge. Therefore, thanks are due to many organizations and individuals: among them are the Children's Center of Michigan, especially Dr. Paula Jorné; the Michigan Society for Psychoanalytic Psychology; the Chicago Psychoanalytic Society; the Anna Freud Center (London, England); the Oakland County Mental Health Clinic staff; the Detroit Psychiatric Clinic; the Michigan Psychoanalytic Society; and the Psychohistory Forum.

Dr. Humberto Nagera helped on the original primary paper on China. However, it was my friend, Dr. George Pollock, who, after hearing the paper, and knowing of my additional material, insisted that I should put it into a book, "with just a little bit of extra work." After four years and much more work than anticipated, I produced this volume. With all of the information gathered, I needed an informed, analytically sophisticated editorial opinion. Natalie Altman, who had helped me on an earlier paper, studied my first draft manuscript and apprised me of the enormous amount of reorganization and rewriting I would have to do. This forced me to rethink what I wanted to accomplish. Did I want to publish another scientific study (I already had over 60 publications), or did I want to reach a larger audience, beyond the psychiatric pale?

The answer became obvious to me, as you can tell from my comments in the Preface. Many models come to mind, among them Barbara Tuchman and Oscar Lewis. I would also like to acknowledge a friend who has been a leader, sometimes a controversial one, in the field of psychohistory of childhood, Lloyd deMause. He helped me in the early research phases and was supportive throughout.

This brings me to the difficult project of how to go about putting scientific material into a more widely meaningful and readable form and getting it published. For this I would like to thank Geoffrey Fox, who sent me in the right direction to Plenum Publishing Corporation.

Now began the reworking, rewording, restructuring, re-everything. Plenum (actually Senior Editor Linda Regan and her assistant, Naomi Brier) loved the material, but choked a little on the volume of gruesome detail and redundancy. I cannot thank them enough for their editorial help and support.

But how was I going to handle the volume and complexity of changes needed? Fortunately I had the help of two more special people in the juggling, spelling, and grammar: Jeff Gaydos (an excellent writer in his own right), and Beatrice Breiner (my wife and best critic), who did a Herculean job at the computer. Together, the three of us wrote, rewrote, edited, organized, reorganized, and revised.

Certain organizations have been particularly helpful: The Bloomfield Hills Group of the Greater Detroit Chapter of Hadassah heard a short version of one chapter and gave me a warm and supportive response.

The British Museum, Department of Egyptology and Dr. M. Bierbrier were informative and helpful. He kindly gave freely of his valuable time. Equally generous was Dr. E. Feucht of the Ägyptologisches Institut, University of Heidelberg, who not only gave of her time, but sent me a prepublication section of her book that applied to my area of study. These are two of the world's outstanding Egyptologists.

Another expert outside my own field gave me extensive help in exploring and understanding the vast Hebrew literature. Without that contribution this project could not have been completed. I refer to the Library of the Hebrew Union College in Cincinnati, Ohio. Curator David Gilner has my profound thanks.

But I am leaving out some essential players in this complicated process. Linda Breiner Milstein, my daughter, and a child and infant therapist, made life difficult until I agreed to write the book, then helped by reading and critically evaluating the first draft. Dr. Sam Milstein, son-in-law and medical researcher/consultant, set aside time from his busy schedule to help me make contacts for some of the research. Myles, my son and an M.A. in Chinese history and language, now an attorney, helped me in innumerable ways to understand the Chinese and their history here in the U. S. and when we were together in China. My son Robert and daughter (in-law) Debra have provided help and support that only comes from a close-knit family. Their children, Andrew and Daniel, and Linda and Sam's Noah and Zena, taught me more than all the texts.

Despite all the help I have just acknowledged, it is only fair and just that I take full responsibility for any errors or any difficulty in comprehensibility.

Most of all I want to thank my patients, who have taught me the most. Without their trust I would have little appreciation of childhood and of the child within each of us.

Contents

Chapter 1

Introduction

Those who cannot remember the past are condemned to repeat it.
George Santayana, 1905

The prevalence of child abuse and infanticide in the modern world is not only puzzling, it is shocking. To explain it, many of us tell ourselves that there are "animals" among us, for only animals would be capable of such atrocities. Others blame the stress of work, financial pressure,[1] or violence on television for propagating the abuse of children in our society. But is child abuse and the killing of infants a modern problem—one that only we have invented?

Actually, infanticide and child abuse predate our civilization[2-10] by centuries. They are ancient problems, often more apparent in the great civilizations of our past than they are now. We have been killing, maiming, and abusing our children for as long as our history has been recorded. The question is, why? I believe that to understand this historic legacy of abuse that continues to this day we must step back and compare our society with those of the ancients. We must assume that we are repeating the patterns of human behavior that predate our own time. Our abuse may be modern, but it is abuse, nonetheless.

In this book we look at infanticide and child abuse as it appeared in five of the most complex ancient civilizations: Greece, Rome, Egypt, Israel, and China. We can learn from history; the study of distant cultures can help us comprehend our own, if we use our sources carefully and are wary of making shallow generalizations.

To understand child abuse in each of these five cultures we obviously will look at the way they cared for their children. But that will not give us as full a picture as is needed. Not only is such information often limited, but it can be distorted. To get a clearer view we will look at four additional facets of each of these five cultures. We will examine family life. Clearly, how families relate to each member and between families, and how the state responds to families can tell us about the degree of love and protection held for its children.

Another aspect valuable to explore is the "law of the land." Laws tell us what people were guarding against within themselves, as well as what they valued and wished to protect. For example, a law against infant abandonment tells us of that danger. If such a law is designed to protect the parent's morality, not the child's welfare, we obtain a different picture of that society's attitude toward its children.

The fourth facet, after children, family, and law, is how a culture responded to its most helpless inhabitants; its slaves. Children are helpless, and usually are recipients of the same attitudes directed to other helpless members of a society. And they observe their "slave" caretakers, teachers, and others, and learn about themselves and their parents' attitudes.

The fifth subject of study is perhaps the most important: women. Women are not only producers of children; they are the primary care givers, molders of personality, protectors, teachers, and models for their offspring, particularly in the most formative first five years. How women are treated in a society gives us valuable knowledge about the life of their children. In fact, we will see that the pivotal person in each person's life is mother. Thus, she becomes the essential person to know about to understand and prevent child abuse.

One advantage of comparative social history is that it is less painful to be objective about other people's behaviors than our own. And, by comparing the types, causes, and incidence of child abuse and infanticide in several contrasting societies, we will be able to identify how they are similar and where they differ. This, in turn, enables us to identify the conditions that contribute to the occurrence of these behaviors and their control. Then we may apply them to our own society. Finally, we can begin to imagine how, say, an ancient Greek or Chinese would view our present behavior, what he or she would criticize or praise. This is a powerful technique by which to gain new insights into both their culture and ours.

Can we change? Is it possible to alter the course of human history? We will explore these questions in depth. However, we must first realize that researching family life in ancient times is not a simple task. Despite the breadth of archaeological, anthropological, and historical literature now available, the complexities of each of these civilizations present obstacles to the critic or historian who strives to paint an accurate picture.

Each of the five civilizations we will consider evolved through several periods, during which child rearing and other social patterns underwent substantial changes. Furthermore, family practices differed by social class, especially after the society became complex enough to develop sharply distinct social groups. In Egypt, for example, the marriage and child rearing customs of the pharaohs were not precisely those of the fellahin, or peasants.

Still, it is possible to identify major tendencies in these civilizations, and I will do that while striving for the greatest accuracy based on the available knowledge.

I have chosen the civilizations of Egypt, Greece, Rome, Israel, and China for analysis, not only because they were the largest and most enduring of ancient times, but also because they were among the best documented. But though they left extensive written records, there are still major gaps in our knowledge of their daily lives. We are fortunate that archaeologists, philologists, and physical anthropologists have given us much material for informed speculation. Ultimately, all of our interpretations of the ancient world rely on three types of evidence—historical, archaeological, and anthropological—each of which has its own limitations.

Historical[(A)] evidence is the written record left by each culture's own scribes. The writings of these individuals, however, cannot be considered as either wholly reliable or complete by today's standards. Much of what appears to be history may be little more than fable, even if some slender thread of fact does hold it together. It is also possible that ancient historians may have distorted their accounts to flatter their rulers or, more rarely, to attack them. Perhaps they exaggerated to further their own careers as historians.

Even within the written records, significant gaps exist. For example, little is recorded of natural events and even less of science and the arts. Documentation of the occurrence and effects of human disease is sparse. In more recent, better-recorded history, we know of horrible plagues that devastated entire populations. Plagues and epidemics altered the course of history in medieval and Renaissance Europe. It seems likely, therefore, that disease must have similarly ravished the ancient world. Other types of disease must have ruined crops and killed herds, wreaking havoc in various communities. More importantly, however, for our purposes, is that practically nothing is recorded of the daily lives of the masses of peasants in each society— the large underclass.

We may also turn to the archaeological evidence of ancient civilizations, which depends on inferences about social behavior based on rediscovery of remains of buildings or artifacts. For example, we might be able to deduce data about family size and life if we knew the typical floor plan of a dwelling. Archaeology makes it possible to surmise the size of the populations of towns and their social class divisions. However, the archaeological evidence, although growing with new discoveries, remains limited. For instance, the most important archaeological find from ancient China is the Great Wall, which reveals much about military strategy and perhaps about labor practices, but almost nothing about family patterns. Similarly, much of what survives from ancient Egypt was constructed for mortuary purposes. Though the Egyptian tombs intrigue us with their beauty and hieroglyphic tales, the most accurate information regarding the daily lives of the Egyptians must be ferreted from other sources.

That leaves us with the evidence of anthropological research. This comes not from the remains of the cultures themselves but from studies of similar cultures that are at approximately the same stage of social development. Field studies among peoples who have mastered only primitive technologies and who are illiterate have revealed patterns of belief and behavior that are often startlingly different from our own. These findings can be helpful as we try to interpret ancient rituals we know little about. Yet they are not definitive either. The best interpretation is the one that offers the most coherent explanation of all the available data. By drawing on all three sources— the historical, archaeological, and anthropological—we will try to convey the most complete picture possible of each civilization. Furthermore, we will analyze these civilizations to seek the roots of child abuse using information gained in modern times, from psychological knowledge, theory, and clinical experience.

The five civilizations selected for this comparison were among the most important known to us based on the rich legacy they contributed to the modern world. Themes from ancient Greece, for example, continue to reflect themselves in modern Western literature, philosophy and the arts. Rome, strongly influenced by Greece, has shaped our laws and political concepts, and its language and institutions form an even larger part of the heritage of all the Western countries. The legacy of the pharaohs is still felt in modern Egypt, and that legacy strongly influenced the ancient Hebrews. From the Hebrews the basic beliefs of the three great modern world religions are derived: modern Judaism, Christianity, and Islam. And, of course, the ancient

Chinese are the cultural as well as the biological ancestors of one quarter of the population of the world.

Thus, there are strong connections between us moderns and the ancients; but as we shall discuss in more detail in the chapters that follow, the ancient world fundamentally differed from ours in many ways, even with regard to climate and terrain. For example, in 10,000 B.C. the Sahara was a lush region of lakes and rivers. It did not become a true desert until 4000 B.C. In biblical times the Negev was also fertile and verdant. It is now a desert. The Emek used to be a malarial swamp. All of Palestine, which is now principally arid, had a rainfall so heavy that people used cisterns to collect water, even in the Dead Sea area of Masada. We would not expect, therefore, to find family life similar to that of the desert nomads of later times.

Not only was the land very different in its lush fertility, it also supported far fewer people. The average life span in ancient Egypt was only 20 years, and the total population was only seven million, concentrated in a narrow stretch along the Nile. During the same time the rest of the Mediterranean coast lands probably contained another 15 to 20 million people. During that same period China had a population of 60 million.

These material conditions certainly affected social patterns in numerous ways. For one, with such small populations and short life spans, the physical survival of a culture was more precarious than it is in most places today. A plague, a drought, or a war could result in its total destruction. One would expect, therefore, that each human life would be especially precious. However, that was not always the case.

It is generally accepted, as one scholar[11] of ancient civilizations has stated, that a child in ancient times "was not considered human until certain ceremonies were performed," and only when the child has been "made" human was his or her life sacred and therefore relatively safe. Children who were not thus protected might be discarded in rivers, dunghills, or cesspools, placed in jars to starve, or exposed to the elements and beasts in the wild. The Greek historian Polybius, who was 80 when he died in 125 B.C., blamed such practices among the wealthy for the depopulation of Greece. Besides the killing of children by their parents, child sacrifices were common to many religions of the ancient world.

There is evidence of infanticide in every part of the world.[12-18] It occurred as early as the Pleistocene period[19] (the Great Ice Age) when, it has been estimated, between 15% and 50% of children were killed.[20] The Roman Law of the Twelve Tables is another example.[21] It practically encouraged infanticide, since it forbade the rearing of deformed children. The law also regulated, but did not prohibit, the sale of children.

Infanticide has continued into modern times.[22-30] Despite the many male casualties of war, there were more males than females surviving in Europe until the Middle Ages. This suggests how much more common it was to destroy small girls than boys. Japanese farmers referred to the practice as "thinning out" the family, the same term they used for their rice fields. In India, many daughters were not permitted to live. Eskimos,[31] in times of famine, would leave babies abandoned in the snow, while some tribes of Brazilian Indians would deposit undesired infants under trees. Even in London in the 1860s, dead infants were such a common sight in parks and ditches that they scarcely turned a head.[13,32] In 19th-century Florence, children were abandoned or taken from their mothers and sent to wet nurses while, in the same period in France, thousands of infants were sent to wet nurses in the countryside and never returned (murdered or sold).[33]

L. Williamson,[34] the noted anthropologist, has called infanticide "the most widely used method of population control during much of human history." And we now know that even the practice of separating a child from its mother in the first two years would cause permanent psychological (and even neurological) damage.

Infanticide is commonplace among animals, from the sim-

plest insect to the most advanced primate. It is adaptive behavior, contributing to the survival of the species. In certain
species of birds, for example, the first hatched chick will inevita-
bly kill its siblings. S. D. Hrdy,[43] the sociologist, established
five functional categories of infanticide: "(1) exploitation of the
infant as a resource, usually as cannibalism; (2) competition for
resources where the death of the infant increases the resources
available to the killer or its lineage; (3) sexual selection, where
individuals improve their own opportunities to breed by killing
the dependent offspring of a prospective mate; (4) parental ma-
nipulation of progeny, where parents increase their own lifetime reproductive success by eliminating particular offspring;
and (5) social pathology in cases where infanticide on average
decreases the fitness of the killer" (i.e., disturbed individual less
efficient in coping who can often incur human injury). Human
beings appear to be the only species for which infanticide falls
into the fifth category, social pathology, wherein the infanticide
is for no practical good, not even an imagined one.

In human societies (ancient to present-day), at least in those
that keep good records, girls are killed more frequently than
boys.[36-42] This is indicated by court records and by census data
which show a preponderance of males in various age groups.
Ironically, the only societies that keep such records are those
with a central government strong enough to outlaw infanticide.
A study[43] of infanticide in 84 societies (Renaissance to 20th
century) found that in one-third, children were killed to eliminate defective offspring. Birth spacing was another frequently
cited reason. In 72 societies where the causes of infanticide were
discernible, 36% reported the practice of killing an infant born
too soon after its sibling.

When we speak of "infanticide" and "child abuse," we are
of course using modern terms that would have had little meaning to the ancients. Certainly, if in a particular culture an infant
was not considered human before proper rituals were under-
taken, then killing him or her would not have been considered
murder by the definitions of that culture.

There is also the question of culpability. Perhaps even the ancients would agree that a human being had been murdered, but since one common way of disposing of children was to abandon them in places where they were unlikely to survive, the parent or guardian could claim that it was not he, but the gods or fate that had killed the child. Several myths attest to the belief that it was possible for a child to survive such abandonment—"proof" that fate, or some divinity, favored the child. Among the more famous of the stories of children abandoned to die are those of Oedipus and of the twins Romulus and Remus. Another way of evading responsibility for a child's death was to deprive the child of adequate food. Sometimes enough food would be given to allow survival but in a weakened state, so that any chance disease would likely be fatal. It was then "nature," not the parent, who had done the killing.

For our purpose, we shall define "infanticide" as any death of a child—that is, of a person not yet in puberty—that has been intentionally caused by others, whether by violence, abandonment, starvation, or other means.

It is more difficult to define "child abuse," especially when we look at the variety of practices in ancient civilizations. Sexual stimulation of small children by adults was quite common and accepted in some cultures, and reviled in others.[35] The same is true of corporal punishments. Very often the people administering these treatments did not consider them "abusive," but rather helpful to the growth of the child. For now, we shall adopt a provisional definition: "Child abuse" is the willful infliction of permanent damage—whether physical, psychological, or a combination of the two—on a child by an adult. Of course, the question of what constitutes "permanent psychological damage" is a complicated one that cannot be considered independently of its cultural context. For this reason, the definition offered here is provisional. We shall return to this issue in the last chapter, where we summarize some of the psychological consequences of the child-rearing practices encountered in the five civilizations, as well as those of our own.

Chapter 2

Egypt: The Beginnings

> Hold your tongue in front of your neighbors. One gives esteem
> to the one who knows how to be silent.
> Amenemope, XXI dynasty

We sail the magnificent Nile today and with a minimum of imagination feel as if we have sailed into ancient history. Along the river's banks, where the lush farmlands reach out to the desert, we see scarcely clothed children playing, as their mothers beat laundry against the rocks. The peasant farmers, or fellahin, are irrigating their land with equipment that was invented around the time King Zoser was building the first pyramid, the pyramid of Sakkara, approximately 2650 B.C.

Suppose the day is bright and clear, as it often is, and there is a sense of peace and grandeur, of timelessness. We see native boats, called fellucas, nearby. They are narrow, arched, one-sailed boats and they look today precisely as they were depicted in drawings on ancient temple walls.

In the distance we see the icons of ancient greatness—Luxor, Karnak, Valley of the Kings, the Great Sphinx. The endless deserts extend on either side. The powerful, oppressive sun (Re, Aten) dances lightly on the water. We are at the origins of a great civilization. It is today, but it could be 5000 years ago.

There are many similarities between the Egypt of today and

11

the Egypt of the pharaohs. People are still eating the same basic diet—small amounts of meat, since there has always been little animal life in Egypt and, for the fellahin, the large lima-like bean, "ful," is the staple of the Egyptian diet today, just as it was in ancient times.

In its warm and dry climate, the Nile of antiquity could be depended upon to fertilize and irrigate the land with unerring regularity and abundance. And the same is true today. Through ancient farming methods the fellahin can plant this rich, fertile land and expect produce.

The climate then was hot and dry and relieved residents of housing and clothing restrictions. Today the small children still run naked and housing for the lowest income residents is adequate in its simplicity.

Certainly, the similarities are startling, but then,[1] as we shall see, so are the differences. The male dominates Egyptian life today; he didn't always. When he wants to relax, he heads for the cafe alone. There he can drink tea or strong Turkish coffee, relax, gossip and catch up on the news. Women are not welcome in the cafe. Instead, they visit one another and attend an occasional funeral or wedding.

In modern Egypt, there is a growing middle class which looks increasingly toward Europe and the United States for guidance in dress and standards of living. This newly acquired sophistication is affecting a historically cohesive family life-style—once the strength of the oldest continuous civilization the world has known.

But let us go back. From history[A] we can learn something about ourselves. Let us go back to the origins, when life along the magnificent river was simple, secure, and peaceful.

Because of its fortunate geography, Egypt was protected from the outside world. There was little chance of invasion from even the nearest neighbor, since the populace was shielded by the large deserts to the east and west, ocean and delta swamps to the north and mountains and deserts to the south.

Egypt, the lotus flower, has a stem (the Nile), with a band of fertile land from one to 50 miles wide on either side, flowing down from the south (Sudan) to Lower Egypt in the north, where the flower (the delta) pushes 130 miles wide as it empties into the Mediterranean. Inland, there are five widely scattered oases—outposts, that served as bases for soldiers who could guard against attack.

History and geography are intertwined. There are two Egypts: the Egypt of the Nile river valley and the Egypt of the delta. Even more historically significant are the two Egypts— Upper and Lower, which have always thought of themselves as separate. The symbol of the pharaoh—the double headdress and the double scepter—is the symbol of Upper and Lower Egypt unified as one land.[2]

Because of the Nile's dependability for supplying food and fertilizer, ancient Egyptian life encouraged large families (ample food) and discouraged a need for slavery or mechanization. The limited wood supply determined that their governmental and religious buildings would be stone and that cooking would be simple and brief. The ancients used grasses and dung as fuel.

To understand these people and their culture we need to take a closer look at the general history of Egypt, which is usually recorded in terms of its dynasties. The predynastic period lasted from 4500 to 2920 B.C. and the early dynastic period from 2920 to 2575 B.C. the first intermediate period was from 2134 to 2040 B.C., the second intermediate period from 1640 to 1532 B.C. The New Kingdom lasted from 1550 to 1070 B.C., the Third Intermediate Period from 1070 to 712 B.C., the Late Period from 712 to 332 B.C., the Greco-Roman Period from 332 B.C. to 395 A.D., made up of the Macedonian Period and the Ptolemaic Succession from 304 to 30 B.C., followed by the Roman conquest.

These dull figures do not illustrate the true, colorful history of the West's longest established civilization. The flow of more than 4000 years—a geographic flow of a fertile and increasingly narrow area which therefore brought people into close proximity; a flow of two separate organizational areas, the Delta region and the river region, the flower and the stem; and the flow of Upper and Lower Egypt and its two distinct cultures and ethnic groups. This flow was upset only by the rise and fall of various dynasties, and during occasional periods by turmoil and deadly warfare. By and large, despite these disturbances, what emerges is a period of relative consistency in ancient Egypt. For our purposes, as we glance at the history of this civilization, we will turn most of our attention to family life—particularly, the treatment of women and children in this culture.

The people of Upper Egypt, Nubia,[3,4] were always a well-organized group who lived in two sections, Upper and Lower Nubia. They were unified and nationalistic. Perhaps very early in its history, the organization of Egypt in the north (Lower Egypt) came from near the Delta region; but the total unification of Egypt usually had its origin in Upper Egypt from Nubia. Archaeological studies and radiological examination of skeletal remains of various pharaohs indicate this was essentially a black ethnic group.

Egyptologists[5,6] know that despite their great concern about death and mummification, the ancient Egyptians tended to be lighthearted and fond of life. They supported a basic equality between the sexes and, as compared with other civilizations we will study, responded with equal warmth and tenderness to daughters and sons. This is confirmed through stories and court records where men and women were regarded as equal when it came to proprietorship and competency.

Women were secure in Egypt.[7-12] There was no anxiety about food,[13] shelter, or clothing, and family life was strong and stable. In the history of Egypt we find little evidence of routine child abuse, infanticide, and little evidence of wife abuse.

In this stable atmosphere, family life flourished. The relationship between mother and child was strong. Mothers carried their babies in pouches or slings against their breasts, so their arms could be free to do their work and so the child would always be close by. Listen for a moment to the scribe, Any, as he writes about the devotion of Egyptian mothers to their children: "Repay thy mother for all her care for thee," he wrote. "Give her as much bread as she needs, and carry her as she has carried you, for you were a heavy burden to her. When in due time you were born she still carried you on her neck and for three years she suckled you, nor did she shrink from your dirt."

Both parent and child were comfortable with their bodies. In the warm climate, children remained essentially naked for much of their life and only at puberty did they wear any kind of clothing; a loincloth and belt for a boy, a dress for a girl.

According to the ancient historians[14,15] Diodorus and Strabo, it was firmly established in the Egyptian ethical code that all children born to Egyptian parents must be fed. Child abandonment and child murder only rarely occurred. One mythological anecdote describes the Egyptian feeling toward children. It tells the story of the Greek mercenary, Menelaus, whose life was not going well. To influence the gods in his behalf, Menelaus took two children of Egyptian parents and slaughtered them as a sacrifice. As the tale goes, the Egyptians were so incensed about this that they forced the Greek to flee Egypt.

The Egyptian esteem for children[16-19] wavered only during times of unrest—during invasions, for example, when historians have found descriptions of child murder and abandonment. That kind of behavior was against the Egyptian *maat*, the "soul" of their existence. Mistreatment of children was considered inhuman.

Prior to 1000 B.C., infanticide[20-24] was rare. Parents were required to raise every child they bore, and if they killed a child, they were required to hold the dead child in their arms for three days and nights. Egyptian literature illustrates how men gave special care to their children, and, perhaps, indulged them. There is strong evidence of fatherly love for the small child. The inscription at a royal grave at Amarna tells the story of a premature death: "I was a small child . . . young in years. All friends are grieving, my father and my mother wish to die, my brothers bend their heads to their knees (in grief)" said the son of Petosiris and begs in his prayer "for your Ka. . . small child, whose lifetime ran out all too quickly, so that he could not follow his heart on earth."

Certainly, family life in ancient Egypt did not always run harmoniously. There are references to fathers who behaved cruelly toward their children. Baleb, a thief, abused and raped married women, and after many beatings managed to alienate his son: "His son fled from him to the place of the doorkeeper and swore by God, 'I cannot stand it anymore by him.'" Another story describes the misery of two small children whose mother died when they were still small and who were driven from their home by their father on the day of the mother's death because he took in another wife. An ancient manuscript[25] which is now held at the Leiden museum in Germany describes in dramatic terms what happened to children during "times of unrest." Children of princes were thrown against the walls or thrown into the street. Unwanted or accidental children were abandoned in the rocky desert. Aristocratic ladies traded their children for a bed, because they had run out of money or were hiding from the enemy, and small children said: "He, God, should never have given me life."

The Egyptian was conscious that there was right and wrong,[26] and did not accept infanticide, as was the custom in other cultures during that era. Thus, a letter from Hilarion to his wife Alis from the first century B.C. indicates a Greek custom (Ptolemaic) rather than an Egyptian one: "When you deliver a child, and it is a boy, let him live; but if it is a girl, abandon it." This kind of hostile preference of boys over girls has not been proven in ancient Egypt. Papyri from the 22nd to 23rd dynasty, which probably were meant as talismans for young women, expressed the wish that either a male or female result from an uncomplicated birth and that the child live. It is, however, remarkable that in one case twins were considered to be unwelcome. This probably was more the result of the dangers twin birth posed to the mother than any superstition or dislike of twins.

Despite isolated aberrations, the overall attitude of the Egyptian toward his child was positive. The child was seen as free of sin because it was still naive, and his transgressions were forgivable. In coffin texts, written before his death, the deceased referred to his own lack of knowledge as childlike. This proved his guiltlessness in front of a divine court. The same court found expression much later when Anschnesneferibe, because she committed sins she hadn't recognized until directly accused, compared her own innocence to the innocence of a child. A priest from Achmin, named Pasemedjemiesach, said of himself: "I am young, one who does not yet have faults." This view prevailed during the later era of ancient Egyptian history. In mythology[27,28] Isis accuses Seth of beating her child "whose fault did not exist."

According to Diodorus Siculus,[29] the Greek historian who wrote around 20 B.C., Egyptian law protected the innocence of the unborn child. A pregnant woman, sentenced to death, was not executed before her delivery because the child was not yet graced with intelligence and should not have to bear punishment. Not only the human child, but the newborn calf was considered pure and innocent, as well, which demonstrates a general caring for the newborn.

Plutarch, the Greek historian/philosopher who wrote about Egyptian life around 100 A.D., said the children of the gods had prophetic gifts because of their purity and innocence. The children of Isis were, therefore, able to reveal where the coffin of Osiris had drifted. Other authors describe how children fell into trances during the procession of the Holy Apis bull and gave oracular statements.

Even the orphan was treated well. Egyptians felt a duty to care for him and his mother. A child was an orphan only if it was deprived of its father. This shows how difficult it was for women to take care of their children alone. It also shows that women were considered inferior to their husbands, for their children were called orphans while the mothers still lived.

In the confusion of the First Intermediate Period the poorest people suffered most from the deprivations; as is usually the case, this included the widows and orphans. It is understandable, then, that in literature the care for them is always stressed.

The Egyptian king Mentuhotep stressed child care as among his good deeds: "I fed children with my hands, I salved the widow" and "I have raised a child and buried the old ones." He gave his son this advice: "If you are given a list of the gifts a poor man made to a widow and to an orphan, diminish his taxes to a fraction of the usual so that the one who fell into bad times may be able to breathe."

Amenemhet I boasted, "I gave to the lonely and raised the orphans." The nobleman Meheri I mentions twice how he took care of the orphan child. He "saved the widows, supported the needy ones, buried the old and raised the children." Further, he emphasized, "I allowed the widows to breathe who had no husband, I have educated the orphans who had no father."

On a stela—the inscribed stone near a grave—the person who died praised himself for being one of those who "buried the honorable old people and kept the children alive." According to other inscriptions, the lot of widows and orphans lay in God's hand, making it clear that the loss of a father or husband was so catastrophic that God was the only alternative as provider. "Because you are the father of the meek ones, the husband of the widow, the brother of those who are rejected and the protector of those who have no mother."

Even if it was the duty of the kings, privileged noblemen, and persons of wealth to take care of orphans, many did not uphold their responsibility. Many orphans roamed the streets freely. "If one throws one's lot with God," so it says, "many an orphan will have taken care of himself." The metaphor "but when the homeland is far, the head is bent in sadness, like that of an orphan on the periphery of a strange city" refers to vagrant homeless children. Trial records indicate that many of these children were uprooted in this way.

The attitude toward the illegitimate child appears to have been less positive. It was apparently immoral, if not punishable, for a single woman to have a child. However, according to Diodorus there were "no bastards" in Egypt. The children of the secondary wives of a man in ancient Egypt were not considered to be bastards because every father was known.

From earliest historic times small pottery figures[30-35] of naked children have been preserved. The boys, with strongly accented sexual organs, usually squat on the floor and move the fingers of their right hand to their mouth. The girls, with sexual organs rarely depicted, are standing with their right index finger in the mouth, the left arm hanging down alongside the body (or both arms tightly along their body). Figures of women with one or two children in their arms also were found, a number of them in the Temple of Satt on Elephantine (island), others in a cachet outside of the Temple area of Abydos. These were apparently votive gifts, perhaps intended as prayers for protection of the child. The figures of women with twins in their arms indicate gifts of thanks after a safe delivery.

The Egyptian child was breast-fed until his third year or longer. Small statuettes are found of women who breast-fed their children in the field, in the kitchen, during a boat voyage, or while making music. But wives of high officials employed wet nurses who were closely integrated into the family circle. In fact, stelae were erected depicting royal wet nurses with the royal babies sucking on their breast. These wet nurses and their husbands usually achieved high positions. Satieh, for example, became the royal consort of King Thutmose III. She was the daughter of the royal wet nurse, Ipu.

The belief was strong that the milk of the wet nurse bonded the baby to its nurse. Kings were depicted suckling the breast of a goddess. In this way the king would enter into a family relationship with the goddess and be recognized as her son. This indicates the importance of the child and that the wet nurse was part of the family—not a distant employee.

The intimacy of the wet nurse with the family is significant, I think it is similar to the intimacy between mother and child among the fellahin. Since the child's world was and still is essentially the same from culture to culture for the first two years, and generally is quite similar for the first five, whoever is responsible for major contact with the child during those first two years is someone to whom we should give attention. Almost invariably the caretaker was the biological mother, though there were exceptions, as we see here. But if we observe the experience of the child's caretaker, we will also learn more about the environment of the young child.

A woman who possesses self-respect, and who has received respect, is more likely to be well-adjusted. This factor cannot be overestimated when it comes to taking care of a small child. As the main caretaker, her feelings and attitudes are transmitted to the child long before the child has any conception of himself or the world around him. I am convinced that how a child is held and treated by the mother is sensed by the child and helps to determine its security. A mother who is tense has more difficulty giving a general sense of security to a child. As a result the child may acquire lifelong psychological difficulties.

In these and other ways we find that children were important in Egypt's Old and New Empire. For example, in artifacts[36-41] from the Old Empire, growing children were often represented at play. Children were shown accompanying their parents at the bird hunt with a bent stick or, if they were fishing, with fish spears. These depictions become more infrequent during the Middle Empire in times of social change, and increased again in the New Empire, when children are again shown participating in the events of daily life. The girls cry and wail during funeral processions, small children are carried by women or older sisters in their swaddling cloths, boys as well as girls participate in the sacrificial acts for gods or for the dead. When the gold is distributed the children celebrate with the adults.

During their first ten years, children[42-51] were considered innocent, but they had responsibilities and were required to love and honor their parents. Children, too, were honored and respected if they belonged to a higher social standing. When they were initiated into adulthood, a wreath or belt was prepared for the adolescent and circumcision could be performed at the same time. Adults praised the adolescent for his independence and responsibility and, in official families, conferred the first office upon them. Boys studied from their eleventh year, and for the ten years following, the occupation they would practice for life. Ramses II, for example, was promoted to colonel (title only) as a 10-year-old. Though children received their "offices" or titles as youngsters, they required adult supervision. Thutmose III said that his 18-year-old son, Amenophis II, was "not wise." Clearly, then, the juvenile was considered a child, though they were given the titles of office they would later exercise.

However, there was responsibility—even in adolescence. These young "adults" were expected to assist their parents in the transition from life to "life after death," particularly by the final preparation of tombs. Much of the parents' adult life was spent in preparation of their own tombs so that only a modest amount of time and money would be necessary for the final entombment when they died.

Child mortality was quite prevalent in Egypt. For cure of childhood diseases medical incantations, talismans, and dubious drugs were administered. However, the size of the special children's cemetery in Deirelmedineh illustrates the failure of these procedures.

It is evident that the children were well cared for, however, and loved by their parents.[52-59] They were especially distinguished by a sidelock of hair. This special lock of hair can be seen in the depiction of children in various paintings and in the hieroglyphic descriptions. When a child became of age (10 years) this sidelock was cut, indicating the status of adulthood.

There were large families, and, as might be expected, social difficulties, including delinquency. But evidence from this time shows that delinquents were not severely punished; certainly not by death or banishment.

In cases of family debt, the creditor could legally proceed against the children as well as the slaves of any defaulter. Thus the children were not completely free from danger.

Children—boys, as well as a few wealthy girls—were also educated. Schools were attached to the local temple and the priest became the teacher of the wealthy children. The teacher's primary function was to produce scribes who would do the basic clerical work of the state. To learn, students copied texts on pieces of pottery, and only after they had perfected their technique in writing would valuable papyrus be used. Using a rod for beating the child as a disciplinary action was an extensive and accepted part of pedagogic technique.

Though children were disciplined severely in schools, they were appreciated in many ways. They were given toys, and they attended family parties to celebrate with other children. Boys were taught to read and write. They learned the basic morals of their culture—respect for parents, honesty, and humility. Those girls who were lucky enough to be educated were taught to read and write so that they could earn a living as scribes and perform tasks for the personal pleasure of their family.

Many of the students graduated and attended a higher school, attached to the state treasury in the temple. These were schools of government, designed to train civil servants in public administration. Graduates were sent to work with officials who continued their education even further.

Aside from their secular studies, children were taught the lessons of their gods.[60-62] Teachers made extensive reference to procreation, and there was extensive sexual play by boys and girls—including siblings. Emphasis was also placed on excretory activity, particularly defecation. Seeing life coming from feces (flies, maggots), Egyptians believed that feces had sacred and magical powers.

The number of brother/sister marriages[63-70] increased during the Ptolemaic period, but not before and became frequent among wealthy commoners during the Roman period. Incestuous marriages had become so common that by 200 A.D., two-thirds of the middle-class couples in the major cities were married siblings. Egyptian poetry had words for lover and beloved which were identical to the words for brother and sister.

Another important element of ancient Egyptian life[71-75] was the extensive sexual activity required of the pharaoh. He had many wives, though only one "first queen." He also had many "little queens" and concubines. The pharaoh's sexual exploits were so important that wealthier wives of royal lineage would offer themselves to him or one of his princes so that they could announce that their genitals had been anointed by the god pharaoh.

The phallus was honored and vitally important in the religious and cultural life of Egypt. The gods are shown with an erect phallus, and a pharaoh was expected to demonstrate in public that he had one, too. At certain ceremonies, the pharaoh would stand before the people and show his erect phallus. Indirectly, this would be shown many times when his erection would lift his loincloth.

His activity with concubines and little "queens" was intended to maintain fertility in the land and to keep peace among the various nomes (like states or counties) and their nome-archs (leaders), and the royal families of the nome-archs. By producing many children from the royal loins that were part of the royal lines of various nomes, the pharaoh was able to maintain peace in the land. He was also expected to travel annually up and down the Nile, participating in religious and sexual ceremonies at each of the multitude of shrines along the great river. This had to be recorded by various scribes who were witnesses to the sexual prowess of the pharaoh.

Religious[76] prostitution was practiced on a small scale, but not as widely or cruelly as in many other cultures in that part of the world. For example, if a girl from a noble family was consecrated to the god Amon to become a temple prostitute, she would remain there until she was too old to satisfy the gods. She would then receive an honorable discharge from the temple and could marry a noble, where she could once again move among the highest circle in the land.

Of course, sexual activity was not reserved for royalty. Normally, brothers and sisters would have sexual relations[77-81] by the time they were 10 to 12 years of age—about the time puberty would begin in this warm climate—and half brothers and half sisters who were in the royal line would be expected to engage in sexual activity for their experience and training in preparation for marriage. Since the proof of the royal lineage and of property transmission had matriarchal determination, sibling incest and marriage among the royalty was considered reasonable. An ancient Egyptian aphorism indicates how common sisterly incest was: "You can sleep in a woman's bed for 100 years, but you will never know her heart until you care for her as a sister." Children would commonly marry between their 13th and 15th year.

To prepare children for their early introduction to sexual activity, it was common for nurses and wet nurses to play with and suck on the male child's genitals so that little boys would have stronger erections. This activity was known as "playing with the sweet finger" or "little finger."[82]

One translation of various Egyptian papyri reveals the following: "Do not have intercourse with woman (still) a child or . . . with a vulva of a child[83] . . . " We see here, then, that although adults may have tried to stimulate a child's sexual organs, the Egyptian drew a boundary line. Adults were strictly prohobited from having intercourse with a prepubertal child.

Young women were expected to be as active sexually as

young men. Women normally took the lead in courtship, and sexual activity was frequent, and open prior to marriage. The Egyptians did not conform to our definition of modesty. Women were considered modest even when seminude (prior to puberty only), since nudity was acceptable in Egypt's warm and natural environment. However, marital fidelity was widely practiced.

The Egyptian gods[84-89] were highly involved in deviant sexual practices, as well as murder. Egyptian mythology shows that the gods not only participated in incest, but committed infanticide, patricide, and matricide as well. This hints strongly that in the early prehistory of Egypt, the people imitated their gods or created them in their own image and practiced such activities among themselves. In fact, though their tombs do not indicate the existence of widows, widowers, divorcees, homosexuals, or other sexual deviations, it is known from writings that all these phenomena occurred. Stories were whispered about an affair between a pharaoh and a military officer, and there were homosexual episodes in the myths of Horus and Seth.

Homosexuality was common in the soldiers as a group, but it was not their primary sexual interest. The concept was that if you had anal sex with a man, this would alter that man into a woman for that period of time, thus making the man who mounted stronger. He would possess the strength of the man he had "turned into a woman." This also would make him stronger as a sexual figure with women.

The Egyptians, it seems, had a very mixed attitude about sex. They were concerned that there be enough sexual activity and procreation, but they also considered it a subversive force to be controlled. Thus, in their myths, sexual activity was depicted as an evil seductress. In their mythology, a symbol for eroticism was a heavy wig with nudity. In their erotic material, various sexual positions would be shown in which the woman was portrayed as receiving no pleasure from the activity.

The ancient Egyptian lived by strict codes, governed by fear of the whims of their gods. For example, there was such fear of the dead that Egyptians would spend large amounts of money, as well as time, to make certain that the deceased would not be angry with the living. People were devoted to their gods, and in fear of them—including the high priests, who interceded on behalf of the people, and the pharaoh, who was a god himself. As a result, people volunteered to help erect national monuments to appease the gods. These workers were not slaves, but average citizens who labored out of fear and dedication, and because it paid well.

Slave labor[90-97] existed primarily in the mines, quarries, and aboard barges. In fact, until near the end of the dynastic period, the land was so lush and prolific that there was little need for slave labor, though it did exist. Slaves consisted mostly of foreigners captured during battles, who were treated rather well compared with Grecian or Roman slaves. In addition to adequate food and lodging, they received a yearly allowance of clothing, oils, and linen. Their working hours were reduced when the weather was hot, and they were not physically abused. They were also not considered the most lowly members of society. Lower still were the criminals—including officials who had been found guilty of corruption—who, following the removal of their noses to brand them for life, were banished to the frontier fortress of Tjel or forced to labor in mines in the Sinai and Nubia. There were also servants who were semislaves— singers and attendants—women who might well have provided affection and sexual attention to the head of the house.

Recent studies of artifacts indicate a larger middle class[98] than was once supposed. With the existence of a large middle class came an activity that would never have been tolerated in a slave society: strikes. For example, the workers at one construction site went on strike to have their wages paid more promptly, for better working conditions, and higher wages. The strike was a massive and successful undertaking. It involved thousands of workers and the village where they worked. Their main worries concerned low morale and decreased income; they felt unappreciated. The strike was settled peacefully at the pleadings and encouragement of royalty. Afterwards, royal courts were established to hear charges of dishonesty made against work leaders.

Although it is true that Egyptian peasants were exploited by their masters and tax collectors, and were at the mercy of the elements as well, by the Late Kingdom, Greek historians Herodotus and Diodorus observed that the exploited fellahin were still better off than the lowest level of the Greek society.

Until 1000 B.C., punishment for crimes was primitive. Hands would be severed for minor crimes, and lips, noses, ears, and eyes excised. Killing as punishment for minor crimes was not rare, and torture-killing was rather common. The guilty might be embalmed alive. During the same time, any criminal who fled Egypt and was brought back was not only punished for his crime, but his house would be burned and his mother, wife, and children killed as well.

The members of the domestic court (*kenbet*) consisted of local village officers and people accorded special respect in the village. This court had the power to settle all civil actions and could decide very minor criminal matters. Major cases were referred to an advisor at Thebes who worked directly for the pharaoh.

By the fifth dynasty of the Old Kingdom, intricate and precise laws regulated private property. There was absolute gender equality before the law. Torture was only used occasionally. Beatings with a rod, mutilation, or exile to the mines, which often led to blindness and death, were more frequent punishments. Guilty criminals, masters who beat their servants, or taxpayers who refused to pay were often beaten on the soles of their feet.

The Egyptians did not have a true police system and, until the beginning of the 18th dynasty, their army was always small. The greatest control of the people was through fear of their gods.

In the laws of ancient Egypt, equality was due everyone—justice for all. In fact, all government officials were expected to learn the following text: "See equally the man you know and the man you don't know, the man who is near you and the man who is far away."

It is important to remember that Egypt's cultural and technical development occurred in virtual isolation. The origin of their language was originally Semitic, from western Asia, and used pictography; but they went on to develop their own form—an ideography—because their ideas became too complex for simple pictures. By 1000 B.C. they developed an alphabet of 24 consonants which later traveled from Egypt to the Hebrews, and via Phoenicia throughout the Mediterranean. (For comparison, at this period of time the Chinese had a dictionary of 40,000 characters.) It has become our basic alphabet (from the Hebrew, "aleph bet," the first two letters of the Hebrew alphabet). The Egyptians themselves never fully adopted the alphabetic form of writing. They mixed their alphabetic writing with pictographs, ideographs, and syllabic signs. This mixed type of written communication was used to the very end of their civilization.

On the more technical side, clocks were developed by 1500 B.C. The famous Roman architectural form of the arch was obtained from the Etruscans, who took it directly from the Egyptians.

From the end of the Old Kingdom until the early period of the Ptolemies, 50 pharaohs erected temples at the great religious city of Karnak. This massive aggregation of temples covers 60 acres and is one of the most magnificent creations of man. They created a remarkable culture—one which despite the looting and destruction of man, is still impressive to even the most unsophisticated eye.

Since Egypt was not dependent on external trade for its food supply or any other basic requirements, everything the citizenry had they developed themselves. They fermented grain, leavened bread, and learned to preserve fish and poultry by drying it. The Egyptian peasant was adequately fed with bread, beans, beer, and onions and occasionally fish and eggs. The wealthy Egyptians ate more eggs and a variety of other foods, including fowl, honey, and milk.

Although the Egyptians were self-sufficient and remarkably developed for an ancient culture, many naive beliefs prevailed, such as the earlier-mentioned reverence for feces. Not only was it considered important in the fertilization of the land, and as fuel, but it was seen as the source of new life. Egyptians saw insects appearing and flying from dung. They therefore believed that dung could produce new life. They saw the dung beetle make small pellets of dung and roll them away to its nest, and from the dung ball would come new dung beetles. The dung beetle became an important figure in the Egyptian pantheon of gods, and fecal play became an important part of the culture. This, of course, inhibited a hygienic way of life and contributed significantly to the prevalence of disease. Still, though they were captivated by feces and the dung beetle, Egyptians still kept themselves cleaner than their neighbors in such surrounding cultures as Libya and Syria. They washed in the Nile several times a day—at daybreak and before and after their main meal. They also differentiated between clean and dirty water and had techniques for water purification.(99)

The ancient Egyptian worshiped the Sun (Re) and gods related to it (Horus the Hawk, Night, Moon). In addition, gods of the Nile were worshiped as were animal anthropomorphic gods. Sometimes animals themselves would be deified and women would be offered to these animals as sexual mates, particularly the bull as an incarnation of Osiris. By 1000 B.C. this activity was not rare and women were sometimes offered in coitus to a bull or a goat.

The phallus was important for all the male gods. It is interesting to note that male animal gods received female humans for coitus, but female animal gods never received males. By our standards, then, women were denigrated and the phallus of the man worshiped.

Egyptian religion and culture held no concept that God and mankind were related; man was insignificant. Egyptians would bow down in front of a beast/god. Men throughout their lives were in bondage to the gods and pharaohs. Human life had less value and many thousands were sacrificed for the good of the nation and the gods. The Greek historian Herodotus observed that in the time of Pharaoh Necco II (609-588 B.C.) 120,000 laborers were worked to death in the construction of a canal connecting the Nile to the Red Sea.

Central to the Egyptian religion was the concept of the solar cycle in which the sun god, Re, is born anew each morning, sails across the sky, ages, and dies. He travels through the underworld to be regenerated each morning in a birth out of the anus or the vagina of the sky goddess, Nut.

Egyptians believed in an afterlife—a series of adventures and struggles preceding a day of judgment, when a person's past was weighed in balance against Ma-At, symbolized as an ostrich feather or as a goddess with a feather. Thoth, the scribe god of wisdom and justice, performed this weighing operation before the god Osiris, who presided with 42 others. If the heart and Ma-At were of equal weight, the person would be presented to Osiris in triumph to join the gods. Those failing the test were devoured by a female hybrid animal monster, known as "Eater of the Dead." This shows a strong negative attitude toward women.

Egyptians believed that everyone, male and female, had a double—a "Ka." The Ka had a life of its own which would be preserved much longer if the flesh could be preserved. Thus, mummification, and the building of pyramids as special tombs to preserve and protect the body, became a focus of Egyptian culture. The tombs were prepared so that the Ka in the afterlife would have the food and implements it needed to survive. The Egyptians wanted to provide well, not only for themselves, but also for their dead.

Certain aspects of the Egyptian family[100-107] showed a tendency toward equality of the sexes. Evidence from a stela near a burial site shows that a man's wife and children as well as his parents and grandparents are represented. In fact, the mother is shown more frequently than the father. Women also had special rights as wives; normally, a man had only one. She went about freely and was not restricted, as women were in other parts of the Middle East. A marriage contract was essentially an economic pact that formalized financial arrangements made at the time of the wedding. Its main purpose was to keep the property in the family. Though property descended through the female line, for practical purposes, the property was controlled by the men. If a couple divorced, the husband was required to turn over to his wife a substantial share of the family property, unless he could prove adultery. At the time of a wife's death, the inheritance went to her child, and there was a marriage contract that determined the dispensation of family properties. She could also write a will, and dispose of her property as she wished.

Comparatively, then, the Egyptians showed an advanced attitude toward women.[108-117] Though a man was permitted more than one legitimate wife, it was rare that he would marry more than one. Royalty and the very wealthy were the exceptions.

In the various tomb paintings the wife is shown accompanying her husband during feasting, hunting, and other significant activities. In expressions denoting the wife, the husband's name is often coupled with hers, as in "his beloved wife, his darling." The pharaoh Ptah-hotep wrote, "If thou art a man of note, found for thyself a wife and household, and love thy wife at home, as it beseemeth. Fill her belly, clothe her back; unguent is the remedy for her limbs. Gladden her heart, so long as she liveth; she is a goodly field for her lord."

More evidence of the importance of women in Egypt is found in the Old Kingdom and Second Intermediate Period. During burial arrangements royal ladies were given prominence, and did not merely accompany the royal male. A term for a female scribe was noted in the Middle Kingdom and, in the Late Period, graffiti in the Step Pyramid refer to the literary efforts of women.

Important papyri now preserved in London and Paris museums offer good evidence that many marriages were arranged by parents or a third party. However, the young people did enjoy freedom in romance and often helped their parents arrange the proper marriage for them. Lovers would commonly use the term "brother" and "sister" when referring to each other. This obviously refers to the sexual freedom prevailing between brothers and sisters, but did not necessarily denote an incestuous marriage.

A common depiction of the Egyptian family shows father and mother holding each other by the hand or about the waist. The youngest and smallest of the children is close to the parents. Royal couples are shown in loving poses and described as being openly affectionate.

The scribe Any (Ani) advised people to marry young and have plenty of children. As many as 15 children in one family— not necessarily from the same mother—was not rare. This, of course, would indicate little infanticide, but it does not deny the strong desire of every Egyptian to have a son. Even with 15 daughters it was a calamity not to have a son, because boys were needed as participants in religious ceremonies involving the preservation and entombing of the parents. As in so many cultures, it was a son's duty to keep his father's name alive.

Despite their propensity for large families, the Egyptians developed methods of birth control.[118] As in the case of the Greeks and the Romans, most of these methods involved only the female. The chief contraceptive methods of the ancient Egyptians were ovariotomy, prolonged lactation, and herbs and chemicals with tampons.

Despite the relatively liberal attitude toward women in Egypt,[119] there were occasions when women were clearly abused. It was a common occurrence among workmen to "assault strange women," any not part of the community nor belonging to a particular man. Ramses III prided himself on making it possible for women to travel on the roads without fear of being assaulted, indicating that prior to his reign, and probably during the intermediate period of anarchy, such travel was unsafe.

The primary role of women was to raise the children, decorate the home, and decorate themselves for their husbands. Unless there were servant girls, women were expected to stay home and do the menial tasks around the house. Extensive housekeeping was not required because of the climate and simple dwellings. The larger homes would have many servants to do household chores. Women were also expected to guard themselves from the sun and in northern (Lower) Egypt, they prided themselves on being fairer skinned than the darker women of southern (Upper) Egypt.

By the time of the New Kingdom, women's status had improved and they were more prominently engaged in community activities. The Late Period restoration by the Nubians saw a return to their earlier, more restricted position in life. Women usually did not hold any important leadership positions with the occasional exception of some priestly functions. A few royal women also had political power. In fact, the queen Hatshupset declared herself a male god and wore a false beard and phallus. But a woman's most common title was "mistress of the house."

Except for the few wealthy women who were sent to school, most were illiterate and were thus barred from the bureaucracy and from participating in the intellectual development of the community. Men were respected for their age and wisdom—particularly if they were obese. Women, on the other hand, were expected to be slender.

With all its rules, the life-style of the Egyptians was not necessarily respected by outsiders. In fact, Romans and Greeks criticized the Egyptians, especially for the relative freedom they allowed their women to enjoy, and for their abstention from infanticide. The Greeks and later the Romans were surprised that the Egyptians did not remove what they considered "unnecessary progeny" from their society. Apparently the Egyptians could not understand the Roman and Greek attitude, either.

We shall see that some of these basic differences in opinion and approach will tell the story of the varied development of other ancient cultures—especially in terms of the treatment of children.

In summary, the Egyptians had a family-oriented society. They followed a basic system of matrilineal descent and inheritance. Union between close relatives was customary and considered suitable. The status of the wife was much higher than in the ancient cultures of Greece or Rome. Women shared recreation and work with their husbands, but they were never considered absolute equals. A wife could divorce her husband, with similar freedom and penalties as the husband. Parental power over the life and death of a child was not exercised. Exposure of infants and the premeditated murder of children for purposes of economy were considered vile acts. Both father and mother were responsible for their children's education. Lastly, the kings (pharaohs) were gods in a theocracy, with an extensive involvement with death (necromancy) in their religion. Egypt, though at times perverse by our standards, was a comparatively healthy civilization during times when others were far worse.

Chapter 3

Greece: The Heights and the Depths

> *Whenever the number of those in the middle state has been too small, those who were the more numerous, whether the rich or the poor, always overpowered them, and assumed to themselves the administration of public affairs. . . . When either the rich get the better of the poor, or the poor of the rich, neither of them will establish a free state.*
> Aristotle, 334 B.C.

We enter ancient Greece from the mountains, with a deep appreciation for the brilliant beauty of the land and sea. We arrive with a shepherd, who is dressed simply and leads us across the verdant hillsides with his sheep. By daylight he is at ease. When night falls he must worry, for the hills are also home to wolves and bears, and his sheep are their prey.

We leave modern Greece of the present with its sophisticated cities and return to an earlier period. Across the valleys below us are small, prosperous farms—each separated from the next by a pile of stones that differentiate one from the other. It is 800 B.C. and the scene is more pastoral. As we close in, we see a town with low, flat buildings, one or two large temples, and a steady flow of pedestrian traffic on the streets.

We enter the town and see slaves, dressed in rags, sweating in the Grecian sunlight under the burden of their heavy labor.

It is early in Grecian civilization. Its greatness and its ultimate decay are at present beyond imagining.

Geography[A]

In ancient times Greece was a conglomerate of coastal and mountain areas made up of a series of islands in the southeast corner of Europe. It occupied the southernmost part of the Balkan Peninsula and included numerous islands in the Ionian and Aegean seas. Mainland ancient Greece was divided into two sections by the Gulf of Corinth. In the North were the regions of Attica, Boeotia, Epirus, Thessaly, and the peninsula known as the Peloponnesus. In the Aegean Sea were the Greek archipelago, the Cyclades, and the Dodecanese islands.

Greece is mountainous, divided by narrow, swift rivers, with some small fertile valleys. In ancient times barbarians lived beyond the mountains. In the 8th century B.C. Greece was heavily wooded, but the forests were stripped for lumber late in the Roman period, around 200 A.D.

Ancient Greece was predominantly a self-sufficient agricultural society, with a large production of grains, olives, citrus fruits, figs, and nuts, and an advanced viticulture. Sheep and goats were plentiful. The Greeks had rich mineral resources in iron, gold in the eastern provinces, and silver in the Athenian mines of Laurium.

Since the demand for wood soared, for use in buildings and ships, the fertile hillsides and valleys were denuded. By 500 B.C. the small farms succumbed to large landowners who raised crops for export, especially olives and grapes. This resulted in less food for the average person. In fact, by 600 B.C. food had to be imported into Greece for the first time, and within 50 years there were many instances of starvation.

Barley was the primary grain, and the Greek's main diet was a combination of gruel and unleavened bread. Leavening was too expensive, so the masses ate the simplest fare. Wheat did not become a product in extensive use until after 400 B.C.

Athens' main exports were silver from the mines of Laurium, olive oil, and later, wine, which was exported throughout the Mediterranean until the Greek and Roman city-states on the Italian Peninsula developed a better wine. Date palms did not grow on Grecian soil, but the fig grew well, and became the staple food (along with olives and grapes).

The very early Greeks (Achaean) were seminomadic and lived mostly on meat. By the time of the Grecian city-states, neither meat nor fish were frequently consumed, except by the wealthy. The main diet was barley (gruel/cakes), figs, olives, and a watered wine.

The civilization that was ancient Greece was influenced from all sides—from the most refined civilizations of the Mediterranean world to the west and south, to the barbaric and primitive elements from the mountains to the north and beyond into what is today Eastern Europe. Beginning in 4000 B.C. the Egyptian and Mesopotamian influence was felt in the islands of the Mediterranean, primarily Crete—so much so that the Cretan culture was essentially Egyptian by 2500 B.C.

The roving pirates of the Eastern Mediterranean, the Mycenae, conquered the people of Crete, intermarried with them, and established a civilization of their own that never reached the pinnacles of pre-Mycenae, Crete. Though there was extensive intermarriage and intercultural exchange on Crete, it remained essentially Egyptian in quality. However, some of the advances of Mesopotamia, Assyria, and the barbaric elements of Mycenae were also evident. The Mycenaean pirates were powerful. With their base on Crete, they subjugated the peoples of the mainland and were paid tribute, including gifts of pubertal-age boys and girls of royalty as human sacrifices to their bull god (a barbaric continuation of the bull worship of Egypt). These children were tied to stakes so that they could not escape when the bull ripped into them.

Between 1500 and 1000 B.C. we see the beginnings of the first primitive Greek alphabet. (Crete, for more than 1000 years, had a written language and a decimal system.) Troy (northwestern Asia Minor) was destroyed in the Trojan War of 1193 B.C., and then the Dorian barbarians invaded and conquered all of the Peloponnesus.

Shortly afterward the culture of Crete was destroyed by earthquakes, civil wars, and an invasion by the Achaeans, who turned it into a vassal state. Phoenician script was introduced into the local simple Greek writing with the addition of vowels by 1000 B.C. In mainland Greece paganism was at its height. The culture was years behind the rest of the civilized world when it introduced the use of iron in approximately 900 B.C.

At the same time Cretans and Phoenicians who had escaped from the Achaean bloodletting established an important colony in Cyprus which maintained its separateness from the Greek mainland (where the Dorians had completed their conquest). The Dorians were originally from Eastern Europe, the area that is now Rumania and Hungary, and left under pressure from the Huns and Tartars. They were among the most primitive, barbaric, and sadistic people in the history of that part of the world. They intermarried with the Greek mainlanders and became an important force both genetically and culturally. By 800 B.C. these new Greek people were an admixture of Cretan, Mycenaean, Achaean, and Doric. They were well organized and had become powerful seamen, having learned sailing from the Phoenicians. They voyaged throughout the Mediterranean, and in a conquering spirit set up colonies all the way to the coast of Spain.

They were also frequently attacked by invaders who came to Greek lands and found no unity in the forces that opposed them. In their entire history the Greek city-states could rarely join in arms to fend off a common foe. Instead, they battled among themselves. Even during the Battle of Plataea in 479 B.C., the Greek army fought not only against the Persian invaders, but against many contingents from Greek cities who enrolled themselves in the Persian cause.

From 800 to 500 B.C. the Greeks became increasingly powerful and spread their culture and colonies across the Mediterranean even into Egypt itself. From 800 B.C. until Alexander's conquest there were 158 major Greek city-states, and probably 1000 more that were smaller. Together they were known as "Magna Graeca."

Athens had been destroyed by repeated wars, particularly with Sparta, so that the Athenian culture had to be literally reestablished by Pericles from 500 to 450 B.C. Earthquakes destroyed Sparta at the height of its military power. The Persian invaders were finally defeated in the Battle of Marathon, and by 400 B.C. the incessant wars between Athens and Sparta brought such massive destruction to Athens that it was never able to return to its former glory. From 352 to 335 B.C., Philip II of Macedon gradually conquered all of Greece, and in fact was welcomed by one faction (aristocrats) of the Athenians as a savior, while hated by another (general citizenry who were trying to get a more equal share from the aristocrats). Philip's son, Alexander (356-323 B.C.), was more Hellenized than his father and more accepted by the Greek people. But he left them to conquer Persia and soon became more Persian than Greek. Alexander used his influence to spread Grecian and Persian culture throughout the world, from India to Egypt.

When Alexander died, his two generals, Ptolemy and Antiochus, divided the empire in half. Ptolemy took Egypt and tried to reestablish the decaying Egyptian culture by appointing Ptolemaic pharaohs. Antiochus took over Assyria and the eastern half of the Persian Empire. The two virtually ignored the Grecian mainland, which later fell to the Romans.

Life in Ancient Greece[1-14]

To understand Greek society, particularly Athenian society, it is important to comprehend the concept of *oikos*, "the family," which is comprised of four basic elements: the male, the female, the servant (slave), and the children. An *oikos* was incomplete without children. The *oikos* only existed as long as it could provide a livelihood for the family unit. If it could not, and there were several sons and daughters, some of them would have to leave home so that the family unit could regain its financial stability. If the family unit was not financially stable, it would lose its position in the larger group of the clan, known as the *genos*. There was no community, or *polis*, in ancient Greece without there being a *genos*, and to be part of a *genos*, an *oikos* had to be intact. Thus, membership, voting rights, and freedom were based on an intact family unit. The son of the house was obligated to marry and produce an heir to continue the *oikos*.

This family-based system accounts for much of the instability and political disarray that existed in the colonies of the city-states, which were populated by people who had left their *oikos* in an attempt to establish their own families. Thus, the city-states and colonies outside of mainland Greece were never as cohesive as those on the mainland. On mainland Greece, individuals formerly were irrevocably tied to their families, but new laws were drawn to begin to emancipate them. (The Macedonian monarchy under Philip swelled the tide of this emancipation, particularly after Alexander.) Thus, pre-Macedonian Greek society was tied to family, the head of which, the *kyrios*, functioned as a governor, ruling over the slaves, women, and children.

By the 4th century, prior to the conquest of Greece by Philip of Macedon, the number of Greeks in the most enlightened strata had declined (due to wars and infanticide) and were governing less efficiently. Revolution of the lower class seemed imminent.

In this period there were more bachelors among the wealthy and courtesans than married couples. Family and society was disintegrating. Since a man had the right to give his property away to anyone he wished if he had no children, a single man without heirs would be fawned over by many sycophants. Those Greek men who enjoyed such toadying would avoid marriage, die without heirs, and distribute their property to their "friends." In the same way men used infanticide to eliminate heirs for whom property would eventually have to be divided.

Prior to this sorry state of affairs, from the Periclean period on, women fell deeper into servitude. A women's function was only to look after her household and produce children—preferably boys. Courtesans (*hetairai*) were educated, while wives were illiterate.

Women of the working class were freer than the aristocracy due to a law passed in 451 B.C. Prior to that time, marriages with alien women had been common enough, but under the new law, children of marriages with non-Athenian women were debarred from citizenship. It was important that all children be born of Athenian women. To prove that they were, these aristocratic women were secluded and ignorant—their chastity therefore assured.[15-22]

The Greeks viewed men as sane and stable while women were considered mad, hysterical, and possibly dangerous and destructive to men. This attitude accounts for the aggressive conflict that was typical of the heterosexual nuclear family in Greece. The Athenian description of women followed their social-medical conceptions of the hysterical character—inconsistent and undependable. One source of this negative view of women may be traced to women's performances in a Dionysian religious ritual, where they fell into hysterical frenzies called "maenadism." The maenads were wild women who roved seminude through the woods tearing apart and eating raw any animal or human they encountered, practices known as *sparagmos* and *omophagia*.

In Athens, a woman's freedom was severely restricted, though she was not impoverished since the property she brought to the marriage always belonged to her. But women were legally without power. A man could sell his daughter or his sister into concubinage if he wished.

In Greek literature (histories, myths, and plays), the mature maternal woman was portrayed as dangerous. In the tragedies, virginal goddesses—young women—were helpful and benign, while the caricature of the mature women shows her as being jealous, vindictive, and destructive. In real life, the older Athenian men often married barely pubescent girls and encouraged them to practice depilation of all body hair—particularly pubic hair. (Clinically, it has been noted for some time that pubic depilation is a response to a phobic problem related to the neurotic notion that the "hairy vagina" can devour the penis— castration by the "vagina dentata," i.e., a vagina with teeth.)

The penis was considered sacred, particularly the glans (head).[23] An exposed glans penis was seen as shocking and awe-inspiring. The prepuce (foreskin) was kept over it, and the penis was often tied with a string called a *kynodesme*, or was closed with a clasp called a *fibula*. Even during the Olympic games when men would compete in the nude, the prepuce would have to cover the glans. For that reason a circumcised male would not be permitted to compete in the Olympic games. Jews of Greece who wanted to be part of the Hellenic civilization would therefore avoid circumcising their sons so that they could participate equally, even though this broke the Covenant of Abraham.[24,25] It is interesting to note that in artworks that depict sexual activities—including an erect penis—the glans is never shown, even though it is physiologically impossible to have an erection with an unretracted prepuce still over the glans.

More evidence of the prevailing attitude toward women can be found in the common "bogey" that was taught to "naughty" children. They were told that the evil spirits were all female creatures. These female bogeys were "Lamia," "Gorgo," "Empusa," and "Mormo." In Greece, there were no bogeymen, but bogeywomen, and these stories added to the Athenian male anxiety toward women.

The attitude in ancient Crete,[26] a culture essentially matriarchal, was somewhat different. There was no evidence that women were restricted to their homes. This was a common limitation in other parts of Greece, where women were not only restricted to the house but sometimes not permitted in certain rooms or areas. The women of the poorer class, who were less protected, were even freer than the aristocratic wives. They left their homes to go to work, and were not confined in the prisonlike manner within of the noblewomen. Even the gods of Crete were more apt to be created in the likeness of women rather than men. Since the death rate was high in ancient times, a great deal of devotion was offered to the female gods of fertility, particularly to the Mother Goddess. In fact, most of the priests in Crete were women.

By our current standards, Crete was a brutal place, but compared with the societies of the Mycenaeans, Achaeans, Dorians, and Hellenes it could be characterized as benign.

Among the early Mycenaeans—barbaric from their roots—there had always been a severe depreciation of women. Women were raped, battered, and generally despised. The Achaeans, meanwhile—though they adopted the Mycenaean speech and culture—established their civilization in Attica under their king, Cecrops. They instituted marriage as a requirement, and abolished regular human sacrifice. They treated their women more equally than the later Athenians. Cecrops required that his people, the Achaeans, worship the Greek gods Zeus and Athena above all others, and this move alone helped to unify that culture, since there were now two major gods rather than many smaller ones. Cecrops' grandson, Theseus, brought Athens to its great power. He ended the sacrifice of children to Minos and other gods, while his grandfather only managed to end the sacrifice of adults.

In a sense, then, it appeared that Greek civilization was

maturing, and though it had become less cruel in some respects, the Achaeans (Greeks) still denigrated literature as being effeminate, and thereby inferior. This gives us some insight into their disdain and depreciation of education and of women.

In Sparta, a cohesive family was discouraged. Husbands were encouraged to lend their wives, if the women were exceptionally strong and healthy, to strong, virile, and brave men, so that they might procreate. A husband disabled by age or illness was expected to invite young men to help breed a vigorous family with his wife.

Only in Sparta was there anything resembling equality of the sexes. A woman had the power—in her husband's absence—to dispose of their real estate as she wished. Also, daughters had the right to inherit property. Since Spartan men were trained primarily for war, and for gathering and controlling slaves, women were left to look after Sparta's economic welfare.

The *kyrios* (father) operated as custodian of the family. Even though he could legally dispose of his ancestral lands, it was considered an enormous disgrace to do so. There was such a concern about the loss of land that daughters, who were permitted to inherit some of the land, were always married to the nearest agnatic relative, such as a father's brother, in order to keep the land in the family. Men who had no natural heirs could adopt sons to keep the inheritance away from their wives.

The main value of the Greek woman was her ability to breed warrior sons. This was particularly true in Sparta. The line between wife and concubine, then, was very fine, and marriage was not a significant religious or legal matter. Marriage was in a sense a *de facto* state. Since there was such a great need for warriors, an unmarried mother of a higher class would be readily married if she produced a strong son.

A woman had the right to marry and have children. In fact, she could demand this of her society. It was very important that the children be legitimate—the children of concubines were aborted, killed, or sold into slavery. This practice of proving legitimacy had two results. It made adultery—the sexual activity of a married woman when that activity was not sanctioned by the husband—a public and a private offense. It also required the Athenians to protect the chastity of their women. Wives were guarded as if they were in prison, and their lives were extremely restricted. Such was not the case for young girls. For example, men were encouraged to participate in sexual activity regardless of the gender of their object of love, and young girls were invited to participate as well.

Sparta, unlike Athens, specified that men should marry by 30 and women by 20. Celibacy was considered such a crime that bachelors would be punished. Such a man might be set upon by groups of women and severely beaten. If a man married and had no children he would be castigated by everyone in the community. A man who did not produce children was a threat to this warlike state that needed soldiers.

Though marriages were arranged by the parents, if an adult was still unmarried several men would be pushed into a darkened room with an equal number of unmarried girls, and by that means mates were selected.

There was no need for adultery in Sparta, for there was much sexual freedom prior to marriage; and husbands were persuaded to share their wives with others, especially with their brothers. Further, women had more freedom to choose mates. Thus, we can see that the position of women in Sparta was better than in other Greek societies.

In Sparta a woman's property always remained separate from her husband's. Though he had control of it while he lived, upon his death this control passed to their children if they were adults, or to the children's guardians if they were minors. While he lived, the husband was responsible to maintain the property and, if the marriage ended without the wife producing any children, he had to repay his wife the value of her original property.

Daughters had an absolute right to inherit their father's

oikos if there were no brothers. But if a father had a daughter and no sons, the best way of preventing the end of the family unit was to find a husband for his daughter and adopt him. The other alternative was to adopt a son of the daughter's marriage. The adopted son or grandchild would then be officially eligible to inherit and sustain the *oikos*.

In Athens, by the time of Pericles—about 475 B.C.—a girl could marry only though parental arrangement. The size of her dowry determined who she would marry, since no man married for love. In Athens, premarital chastity was required of all respectable women, though it was not expected among unmarried men. During the religious festivals there were many opportunities for extensive sexual activity, which was not considered to impair a women's virginal status.

When an Athenian bride went to live with her husband she was cut off from her entire family and became a menial worker in her husband's home. She had no rights of her own and functionally was no longer a citizen. She could not vote. The children she bore were not her own. They were the product of male seed, and she was just the container. All the children came from him and belonged to him. A son could only escape his father's authority once he married. The wife was always under her husband's power and always remained secluded in her house. She could only stay in the women's quarters, and was literally a prisoner in her own home.

In Athens, there was no respect for women, with a few exceptions. In the most primitive Greek communities, at the beginnings of the civilization, some women were venerated as having oracular powers and were considered equal in many ways. It was only as the civilization grew that women became generally despised. In literature there was the image of the young noblewoman, but it was only in the theater that women were actually applauded. In reality they were depreciated and confined to the *gynaeceum*—women's quarters—of the home. Much of the general poetry, except that written by Sappho, is brutal and antifeminist in quality. The love poetry seems mostly written for young boys.

Demosthenes said, "We have courtesans for our pleasure, concubines for our comfort, and wives to give us legitimate children." No matter what occurred, the woman was always a slave to the man. When she was widowed she became the ward of her eldest son. She could never walk unescorted, and was always guarded by a slave. She never went to the market, as this was a slave's activity. In fact, the Greek term for a wife, in Athenian democracy, was a neutral word that meant "object whose purpose it is to look after the household." She was not a person, but a thing.

Pericles was a misogynist and Euripides, the great playwright, was in constant disagreement with Pericles for not hating women. In the great democracy of Athens under Pericles in the 5th century B.C. there were 30,000 citizens out of a total population of 400,000. Of these only 14,240 had full civic rights. The others were children and women.

In the Achaean period (5th century B.C.) children[28-33] were not formally educated, and almost all males and females were illiterate. The Achaeans considered scribes, merchants, and artisans to be inferior, and treated them as such even to the point of enslaving them. They respected warriors and viewed educated craftsmen as effeminate. Education, then, was at best unnecessary.

In Athens there were public schools for exercise, but no true public educational schools or universities. However, there were many private schools that the wealthy could enter. Only a very few Greek women were well educated and most of them were the *hetairai*—the courtesans. An exception was made for certain women who were encouraged to enter the School of Pythagoras, which only operated for approximately 35 years; or the few who studied grammar and philosophy with Pericles' learned concubine, Aspasia.

It is safe to conclude, then, that ancient Greek women were

not only uneducated and despised, but men's revulsion toward them made the ancient Greek male propensity for homosexuality quite understandable.

Compared with other societies, there was extensive homosexuality[34-38] among Greek men. Young boys were often abused. Merchants would import handsome boys to be sold to the highest bidder. They would be first used as concubines and later as slaves. It was considered quite proper for the young men of Athens to engage sexually with older men, and most did. The older man was expected to further the boy's education. (This is true in Athens, but not accepted by some who have studied life in Sparta.)

Thus we can see why Greek literature glorified homosexual love. Both Plato's and Xenophon's symposia presented men who were homosexual. Socrates had homosexual inclinations, but he argued that the physical aspect of it should be minimized. Marriage was never glorified by any of the philosophers. In fact, they often contrasted the beauty of the love of a pretty male child with the tribulations of marriage and the degradation of heterosexual intercourse. Socrates advised Callias to participate more in Athenian government so that he could earn the respect of his boy lover. We can look back on the homosexual pederasty that was so universal in Greek society as a means of "rescuing" the male child from the perceived dangers of women, and training him for the peculiar, unique, erratic ways of Athenian democracy.

Free Athenians began passive homosexual intercourse at about 16, when they began to frequent the gymnasium and wrestling school. For a short period following their military service they would be the active lovers. Sodomy was considered reprehensible to do to older men, but not to young males. Pederasty with a kept lover was expensive and was a habit therefore of the upper class. It was rare for a boy not to have had a male lover.

Sexual abuse was practiced extensively in Crete and

Boeotia, where there were even child homosexual marriages and honeymoons. Boy brothels flourished in every city and a child prostitute could be rented, even at the height of Athenian culture. Older men were encouraged to keep slave boys rather than free ones. Thus, a freeborn child might see his father having sexual relations with a child his own age who was a slave. Male children were frequently sold into concubinage, and sexual abuse of children by their teachers was far from rare.

Homosexuality was a common experience of young pubertal-age boys—as part of their having an older man as a mentor. Usually sex was intercrural rather than per anus. But, being used homosexually was not the first subjugation, degradation, or danger for a child.

In Greece during the 12th century B.C. animals were regularly sacrificed[39-41] to the gods, and on special occasions, to human adults. Human life was considered so short and cheap that there was little concern about killing. When a town was captured the men were automatically killed or sold into slavery and the women were taken as concubines or slaves. The "good man" was one who "fights bravely and dies well." Characteristics such as gentleness, kindness, industry, honesty, and integrity were scorned as effeminate and inferior. This was a society of patriarchal despotism. The male head of the household not only had many concubines but also offered them to his guests. He would slaughter his own children as sacrifices to the gods or simply expose them on the mountainside to die.

There is evidence that "surplus" children—any whose existence threatened family economics—were exposed to the elements and died throughout antiquity.[42-48] Thus the first child of a marriage, whatever its gender, was never exposed if it was healthy. If the second child was a boy, as well as the first, the parents might kill the second boy. And if any more children were born, they were usually killed. There was a fear in the non-Spartan cities that heirs would divide the sacred land. For example, in 6000 families in 200 B.C. at Delphi only 1% had two daughters. So extensive and widely accepted was infanticide that it entered into many of the comedies written at the time and jokes were made about it. In Menander's *A Girl from Samos*, a joke was made about a man who tried to chop up and roast a baby.

It is probable that the poor resorted to exposure more frequently than the wealthy, particularly with those children who were born out of wedlock. Bastards of slave girls, courtesans, and prostitutes were common victims. The most frequently used method of infanticide was to leave the infant in a large earthen jar by a temple where it could be rescued if someone wanted to adopt a child. Otherwise it would die from exposure. Children were thrown into rivers, dung heaps, and cesspools. Wild animals were everywhere. Feeding upon children was part of their sustenance, as Euripides noted in his play *Ion*, "A prey for birds, food for wild beasts, too . . ." In fact, the law required that if a child was not perfect it had to be destroyed. There was even a famous text entitled, *How to Recognize a Newborn That Is Worth Rearing*.

On the tenth day after its birth a child would be formally accepted into the family with a religious ritual and given a name. At this time the child could no longer be legally exposed or abandoned.

In all the Greek cities except Thebes the father had the right to kill his child at birth without question. In all cities except Athens the father could sell his children (even when they were no longer small) to slave dealers. Of course, among the poor, selling children as slaves to pay off creditors was common.

As a result of these prevailing practices, the population of Attica declined. In fact, infanticide was so widespread, and homosexuality and prostitution so pervasive, that the citizen class in Attica decreased from 43,000 in 431 B.C. to 22,400 by 313 B.C.

By the time of the Roman conquest, around 200 B.C., only one family in 100 raised more than one daughter; sisters were a rarity. Families with no children or only one child were ex-

tremely common. A study done in 200 B.C. of 79 families found
that 32 families had one child and 31 families had two. There
were a total of 118 sons and 28 daughters. The infanticide rate
must have been enormous. Cities became deserted and the land
became barren. Family life was disappearing.

A female child not killed by her parents was still depreciated starting with the inferior food she was fed. Xenophon, the
Greek historian and a student of Socrates, wrote that girls were
brought up on a sparse diet with little protein. The girls of
Sparta were reared more rigorously; unlike the boys, they were
not trained directly in the arts of war but indirectly in various
strenuous games. It was emphasized that they become strong
and healthy for easy motherhood and to protect the home front
when the men were off at war.

To keep children from misbehaving and making annoying
demands, parents terrified them with stories about ghosts who
would come and harm them. Warmth was only expressed toward children when they were asleep, and especially if they
died. Children's demands were responded to as unwanted and
unnecessary.

In the more advanced civilization of Sparta the care of children was in some ways inferior to that of the earlier Achaeans.
In a famous story a mother tells her soldier son, "Return with
your shield or upon it." To create a society with such a disciplined soldier class a ruthless eugenic practice was required. A
child who appeared defective would be thrown off the cliff of
Mount Taygetus by the father. To make sure that a child "was
healthy" parents exposed their infants on the side of the mountain. If they survived the exposure they were taken into the
family; but even then they would be placed in uncomfortable
positions with coarse sleeping garments to "harden the body."
By age seven the Spartan boy left his family and was brought up
by the state in a group camp. He became part of a strictly disciplined military regiment. The strongest boy in each class was
made captain and was encouraged to punish the weaker ones,

who in turn were instructed to obey. The purpose of these drills was to create "martial courage," not athletic skills, kindness, or consideration.

All games were played in the nude and quarrels were provoked (by the men) among the boys so that they might develop an even more martial attitude. Bearing pain and hardship silently was required of all. Annually at the altar of Orthia, specially chosen youths were scourged with whips until their blood covered the stones of the altar. The boys would often compete among themselves. The one who cried out first lost the game.

When he reached 12 years of age a boy was no longer permitted to wear underclothing. He was given one coarse garment to wear throughout the year. He could not bathe frequently either, as this would "make his body soft." "Cold air and clean soil" were required to make the body "hard and pure." The boy would sleep in the open all year round and did not live at home with a wife until he was 30 years of age, though he might marry before that, prior to completing his military duty.

His education was so limited that he was barely able to read the basic military text; instead he memorized it. Each Spartan boy was trained to abstain from drinking water so that he could endure living without it for a time. He was also not permitted to drink alcoholic beverages. A Spartan boy was trained for war and for living off the land. He was sent out without food and was encourged to steal to keep from starving, though, if caught, he would be flogged. Those who survived until the age of 30, and did so honorably, became full citizens—an honor not possible for women, since they were not granted voting privileges.

In Athens, until late in history, every citizen was expected to have children. When there were no children, adoption was expected, though, as we have seen, law and public opinion readily accepted infanticide.

In addition to child abuse, another example of Greek cruelty can be seen in their treatment of slaves. In early Achaean culture slavery was not widespread. The land was difficult to farm and the people were not very interested in pursuing agricultural efforts. Their essential source of wealth was the exploits of their warriors, colonizers, and pirates.

Slave labor[49-53] became increasingly important for working the mines. Craftsmen during this period were freemen, not slaves, and although slavery did exist it was not extensive. Most slaves were female domestics, and they were not degraded or abused as they would be 500 years later. The use of slave labor would soon flourish tremendously in Greece.

The institution of slavery is considered a hideous blot on the ancient civilization of Athens. The Athenians themselves knew what the loss of liberty meant. "Half of manhood goes when slavery's day sets in," was a well-known Athenian saying. But they were racial bigots and asserted that because slaves were primarily of barbarian origin, they were slavish by nature. However, the enslavement of Greeks by Greeks was considered an outrage. In Socrates' time a law was passed forbidding the purchase of Greek prisoners of war. But by the 5th century B.C., with the deterioration of Athenian democratic principles, Melian islanders (from a Greek island under Athenian rule) were sold into bondage. Most Greek thinkers, poets, or philosophers of the time never seriously questioned the necessity or morality of slavery.

In fact, no philosophers in all the ancient world, except for the Hebrews, condemned slavery; the greatest philosophers in Greece attempted to justify it. Protestation against slavery was made by playwrights, not by philosophers. In their tragedies and comedies we find the most extensive reference to the unacceptability of slavery. Euripides was the first to denounce slavery on the Greek stage. When Philip of Macedon conquered Greece, he forbade the freeing of slaves because he believed (and rightly so) that this would keep the Greeks weak.

At the height of the Spartan conquest of Peloponneseus, in all of Spartan Attica there were 30,000 citizens, able to keep 120,000 serfs (helots) and 210,000 slaves in subjugation. They could control this vast number of people simply because it had become their chief business. Every Spartan male became a soldier, ready at a moment's notice to suppress a rebellion or fight a war. Among the techniques they would use to control the slaves and helots were regular incursions into the slave population to destroy budding leaders. Thus, because they became a successful slave-managing state, Sparta gave up the human aspect of civilization.

Life was different in Athens. Economically there were three groups of Greeks: the *eupatrides*, who lived in luxury while others did their work for them; the *demiurgoi*, craftsmen and traders; and the *georgos*, the peasants, who worked the smallest and meanest pieces of land and who were usually on the edge of poverty and starvation. Beneath these three classes were the slaves, still a minority in early Athens even among the lower classes of society.

Due to the Athenian ability to rule the seas there was an explosion of the middle class, the *demiurgoi*. The poorest peasant became poorer because he had to borrow money to work his land and the rates were usurious and arbitrarily raised. This made the peasant's small holdings smaller still, and the great holdings of the wealthy even larger. Meanwhile, the middle class expanded and there were no wars to control their expansion. Soon the free peasant laborer had difficulty competing with the slaves who were brought in by the middle class. The growth of slavery dragged the free laborers down to a position of destitution. They could no longer afford to buy produce from large landowners. By 620 B.C. conditions deteriorated to the point that the large landowners began selling their produce overseas. In order to appeal to their new markets they began growing grapes and olives because wine and olive oil sold well in foreign countries.

Soon Athens could only supply the very wealthy Greeks with home-grown produce. The lower classes simply starved.[54] To survive, some Athenians sold themselves into slavery to pay their debts and get some food. Where formerly no Greek would enslave a fellow Greek, least of all an Athenian, this practice now became commonplace.

In 580 B.C. the Athenians made Solon the head of their community and encouraged him to develop a constitution and a "law of the land." He freed all people who had been banished for political offenses and sold into slavery. All debts were cancelled. He also set up laws that greatly limited paternal authority, though he never succeeded in forbidding infanticide. Solon established the most democratic rule of law that had ever existed.

Following the death of Solon (559 B.C.), many of the laws he instituted were sabotaged and destroyed. The laws of Solon (and later, Pericles) had utilized for the first time principles that were part of the Egyptian and Hebrew worlds. But, though much improved, the new Greek legal system was still quite limited. No cross examination of witnesses in a courtroom was permitted, and perjury was frequent. Women and minors could only testify in murder trials, and the testimony of a slave could only be admitted after he had first been tortured. But harsh as was Athenian law regarding slaves, it was so much better than in the rest of Greece that the other city-states began to adopt the "advanced" thinking of Athens. For example, the wanton killing or abuse of slaves was proscribed.

Only in Athens was there any protection for slaves, though they had no legal rights. They could not be severely abused. The rest of the Greek city-states deplored Athenian leniency toward slaves, and viewed it as a dangerous precedent that could lead to a slave revolution.

The Athenians had silver mines at Laurium, managed and operated by slaves, on which they were very dependent, as well as on their olive oil exporting business. When, during the Peloponnesian Wars, Sparta captured Laurium and its mines, the entire economy of Athens was rattled. As a result, Athens became increasingly dependent on slave labor and the economics of selling slaves. Slavery became so extensive in Athens and the rest of Attica that the fate of the entire economy was based on it, and the ancient Greeks lived in constant fear of slave revolts.

In these ancient city-states the vast majority of workers and producers of valued items were slaves. The "democracy" of Greece was supported by only a small number of free democrats—10% to 20% of the population maximum. That meant that 80% to 90% were enslaved.

It seems clear that two factors limited the growth of Greek civilization and led to its decline: slavery, and the increasingly inferior status of women. In the 5th century B.C. in greater Athens, there were 70,000 resident aliens who had no rights and had to pay extra taxes, 200,000 slaves, and a maximum of 130,000 people who were classified as citizens, two-thirds of them women and children, leaving only a small number of freemen.

How could this happen? Slavery was not customary among the primitive Greek tribes that had originally conquered the area. The primitive Doric and Achaean tribes constantly declared war on each other. They usually killed their prisoners or ate them raw (though occasionally roasted). Slavery began when these early Greeks decided to keep a prisoner alive so that he might do some work for them. As the society settled, and commerce increased, they began to sell their prisoners in exchange for commodities. Thus, slavery began as an outcome of war and later the acquisition of slaves became the main objective of war. If a prisoner couldn't redeem himself after a war was lost, he would be sold into slavery. When a city was under siege, the men were usually put to the sword rather than sold as slaves (particularly if the slave market was flooded) and the women and children were sold. In some cities the citizens maintained a certain number of handicapped people, mentally ill, condemned criminals and other unfortunates so that during times of famine and pestilence they could be stoned to death as sacrifices to the gods. Or they might be beaten on their genitals and then burned, and their ashes scattered over the sea as a sacrifice to the gods of fertility or rain.

It is reasonable to conclude that since there was cheap slave labor, there was little urgency to develop mechanical modes of manufacture. Greek scientific discovery was used for philosophical purposes and rarely used practically. There was no demand for technology. When Hero of Alexandria developed the first steam engine in the 3rd century A.D., it was never put to use and was considered a toy.

From our modern point of view, it is difficult to fathom the waste of humanity witnessed in ancient Greek society. But perhaps we can obtain some insight into the attitudes of the people by examining their mythology. Greek mythology[55-57] as narrated by Hesiod was filled with monsters, sadism, and pornography, patricide, matricide, filicide, infanticide, and incest. Uranus, the father, kills all his children except Kronos, and Kronos undertakes (at his mother's behest) to kill his father. The Titans, the siblings of Kronos, help Kronos capture Olympus. Kronos eventually marries his sister, Rhea. But Kronos thinks his children will destroy him as he has destroyed his father. Therefore he slaughters and eats of all his children except for Zeus, whom Rhea has secretly hidden in Crete. When Zeus grows to be a man he deposes Kronos and forces him to regurgitate his children and bring them back to life. He then sends the Titans back into the center of the earth from whence they came. These were the characteristics of the god that the Greeks worshiped.

Some of the quality of Greek life may be understood by analyzing what they idealized. Their great heroic story of the Trojan War (12th century B.C.), written first by Homer (9th century B.C.) and rewritten again and again into the 1st century A.D., characterizes their model for certain human relationships.

When the great Greek horse breaches the Trojan walls, the slaughter begins. There are no heroics at the end of the battle

and no pity for the helpless. Achilles' son Pyrrhus (Neop-
tolemus), "mad with murder," decapitates the wounded Polites
(Priam's youngest son), and when Priam slips in his son's
blood, he too is killed by Pyrrhus. Females of all ages are raped.
Polyxena (Priam's daughter) is sacrificed on Achilles' tomb.
Ulysses (Odysseus) has Hector's young son Astyanax hurled
from the battlements. And it ends in an orgy of murder, rape,
and infanticide while the Greek "heroes" board their ships for
home. What preceded and succeeded this heroic event is similar
in its killing, raping, adultery, abuse, lying, abandonment, family disruption, and lack of human feeling. This kind of violence
is not typical of all epic poetry, nor, for that matter, of all
cultures.

In the religion of the ancient Greeks, the phallus was deified. This was extended later into Roman times with the worship of the god Priapus, who, according to legend, had a large
phallus, and was the son of Aphrodite, the goddess of beauty,
love, and all the sexual pleasures. She was worshiped in a variety of forms in many different cities. Most Greek city-states held
festivals, aphrodisiac, with sexual freedom and debauchery the
rule of the day.

These excesses also characterized Dionysian rites, during
which participants mourned the death of Dionysus, and subsequently celebrated his resurrection in the form of an orgy. This
took place in the spring when the grapevines were blossoming.
The Greek women went up to the hills to meet the reborn god.
While they waited for him they drank and danced in an unre-
strained manner for two or three days, working themselves into
a frenzy and tearing off their clothes. A goat, a bull, or sometimes even a man or young girl would be brought to the rites,
and after varied sexual activity, the women would tear the victim to pieces, drink its blood, and eat its flesh in a sacred com-
munion with their god.

There was also a great deal of phallic activity in early Greek
drama, with demonstrations of Dionysian rites on the stage in

performance of explicit sexual acts. Comedies were phallic, as well, and tragedies included satyrlike Dionysian revelry in which the participants dressed as goats. Goats were part of the mythology and god concepts. They had special aggressive and sexual powers. The word *tragedy* derives from the word for goat song, *tragoidia*.

There was no priest class in Greece and the father usually functioned as priest for the family. The state ruled the priest-hood rather than temple priests ruling the state, as was common in Egypt. In special worship services during times of strife, sacrifices were offered. Agamemnon sacrificed his daughter Iphigenia, and Achilles sacrificed a dozen Trojan youths. The god Apollo required human victims to be hurled from the cliffs of Cyprus, while others would be placed on the altar to die. The Spartans flogged youths to death at the altar of Artemesia. Until the second century A.D. in Arcadia, human sacrifices were made to Zeus.

Even in sophisticated Athens during times of calamity or plague, a well-dressed citizen would represent the community and would be killed in sacrifice—presumably to propitiate the gods. These sacrifices were also practiced during some phases of war as a price for victory. Victorious Greeks would appease the blood lust of the gods by sacrificing someone in the community. When Greece moved from human sacrifice to animal sacrifice it was a significant advance, though the civilizations of Egypt and Israel had taken that step many centuries before.

We can see that religion did not provide the people with much moral support and certainly failed to unify them. Every city-state had its own god. The unifying factor in ancient Greece was athletics—especially the athletics at Olympia. Even war would cease so that opposing armies could support their athletes in the Olympic games. The first true Panhellenic games were recorded in 776 B.C. They became so important that by 476 B.C. athletes from the entire Mediterranean Greek world would enter and compete.

War and killing was a traditional Greek sport. In Greece's many civil wars, the victors would sack the conquered city, kill the wounded, and murder or enslave all prisoners, even captured noncombatants. They would burn the town, destroy the orchards and fields, and exterminate all the livestock. In the most savage of the wars (the Peloponnesian), the Spartans put 3000 Athenian prisoners to death in one foray. The Greeks fought city against city, class against class; war was a way of life. After Greece defeated the Persian King of Kings, they returned home to fight wars among themselves in hundreds upon hundreds of battles. For 100 years after the glory of Marathon in 490 B.C., the Greeks went through a prolonged self-destruction.

Plato revealingly described his Greek compatriots: "They bargain violently in buying and selling, argue every point in conversation, and when they cannot make war upon other countries, quarrel among themselves. They are not given to sentiments; and disapprove of Euripides' tears. They are kind to animals and cruel to men: they regularly use torture upon unaccused slaves, and sleep heartily to all appearances after slaughtering a city full of noncombatants. More or less they are generous to the poor and disabled."

A great deal has been said about the Golden Age of Greek civilization, but it should be remembered that this Golden Age lasted only about 50 years during the second half of the 5th century B.C. This was the period of the flowering of philosophers, writers, poets, sculptors, and architects, and conquests and internecine wars.

As the self-destruction continued, the Athenians hired mercenaries to fight their wars—a milestone in their history, for the Greeks had once been mercenaries in other lands as distant as Egypt. The courts, once just, became corrupt, and city life in Athens became riddled with embezzlement, tyranny, and murder.

Athens began to depend on its empire outside the city limits for supplies. When Sparta destroyed Athens' navy in 404

B.C., the populace became helpless and were unable to provide for themselves. With this decline in Athenian wealth, the price of slaves dropped markedly, yet more slaves were employed in an attempt to meet financial needs.

Because of the extent of slavery in the culture, the Greek ideal had become antimechanical. The artisan was seen as a kind of mechanic. Craftsmen were despised. And except for the writers, poets, and warriors, there was no valid creative outlet for any citizen of Athens.

Thus weakened, Greece fell to Philip of Macedon in 338 B.C. and several years later, to the dictatorship of Alexander the Great. Alexander created the forerunner of the first modern state, putting all the city-states under the control of one supreme leader. Following Alexander's death in 323 B.C at the age of 33, the center of civilization shifted from Greece and became located in Assyria and Egypt.

With the destruction of the family unit in Athens at around 261 B.C., after almost 50 years of war, civilization was almost at its end in Attica. There were so many destitute people in Athens that the unemployed were exported or forced to emigrate. Bands of Greeks roamed the Hellenistic world as small armies of thieves, looting at random, and causing greater disintegration of the Mediterranean world.

Epicurus, a great philosopher and teacher (342-270 B.C.), stands out as a small light in this darkening Greek world. He accepted everyone—women and slaves as well as freemen—into his school and philosophical system. To Epicurus, everyone was equal. Epicurean friendship became the model for future civilizations.

Greece at its height consisted of 158 petty quarreling states involved in internecine warfare. Their political life was, by our standards, not only unreasonable, but absurd. The Athenians chose their judges by lot and their generals were elected in mass meetings.

Each city-state seemed to carry its own philosophy of government to an extreme. Throughout Greek society there existed aristocracy, oligarchy, tyranny, democracy, and even a Spartan military communism. And, there were always slaves. Children were sacrificed meaninglessly. Females were killed as infants, sexually abused as girls, and despised as mature adults. Rightfully, Nietzsche called the Greeks "the political fools of ancient history."

But we find greatness here as well. Greece, in its chaos and cruelty, perversity and inhumanity, produced incomparable masterpieces of literature, philosophy, science, and architecture.

Despite its rise to greatness, the glory that was Greece seems to lose its luster. For with its rise came a "greatness" in the appalling prevalence of slavery, homosexual exploitation of boys, depreciation of women, child abuse and infanticide and, ultimately, the destruction of the family. The glory that was Greece was indeed limited, and exists more in fantasy and historical distortion than in the cruel facts of reality.

Chapter 4

The Hebrews: And God Spoke to the People

> *That which is hateful unto thee, do not do unto another. This is the whole Torah; the rest is commentary. Go and study.*
> Hillel, 50 B.C.

Sunrise makes the rose-colored stones that comprise Jerusalem glow, as it has since King David's time. The sky is clear, the morning brisk but not cold; we leave the cool Judean hills for a very short ride to the lowest spot on earth—the Dead Sea. Here it is much drier and very hot. As we travel along the edge of this strange mineral body of water to En Gedi and Masada we become part of an ancient land. Here where the Dead Sea Scrolls were hidden for over 2000 years we feel the past is now. Forgotten is the narrow passage of land between the Mediterranean and the former malarial swamp (the Emek) now drained by modern Israelis and turned into a lush meadowland. This narrow trade route passage that was such an economic advantage to the ancient Judeans is now a terrible burden since it is dangerously located between the millstones of Mesopotamia and Egypt. All that is now forgotten as we lose ourselves in the past with the seminomadic Hebrews who changed the world.

We enter the world of the ancient Hebrews[(A)] on a desert

caravan in approximately the 12th century B.C.—among the sons and daughters of tribesmen who have been cast out from Egypt, where, for a while, they ruled with the Hyksos, conquerors of Egypt with the Hebrews (17th dynasty, ended 1587 B.C.).

The trip to Palestine has taken decades and settlement is not easy. There are battles and there are losses. But there are victories, as well. Through the years the land is settled, tribe by tribe, though it will not be theirs for long. Because of the power of Palestine's neighbors on either side, the Hebrews are forced to take sides in the struggle between warring empires, to pay tribute to whoever wins and to be overrun.

But their new land is bountiful—truly a land flowing with milk and honey. Even by 100 A.D. it was still described by Josephus as "moist enough for agriculture and very beautiful. They have abundance of trees and are full of autumn fruits, both wild and cultivated. They are not naturally watered by any rivers, but derive their chief moisture from rain, of which they have no want." In these ancient times, heavy rain fills the cisterns and the many wells, which create a network of adequate water supplies for the entire country. The earth is rich, so that when supplied with water it produces abundant crops of barley, wheat, vines, olives, figs, dates, and fruits.[1,2]

It appears that all will be well here, but in fact, the story of the Jewish people is an international tale beset with varying turns of fortune. It is a story in which the people both win and lose, but ultimately it is a story of growth, family unity, and cultural maturation.

We will see that there are some important and subtle differences between the Hebrew concept of one God and the Egyptian god-view. The Hebrews had one God—a noncorporeal God associated with wonder, beauty, love, and mercy. The Egyptian short-lived belief in one central deity did not deny the attendant gods but stressed the one god Aten (Re), who was corporeal. Egyptian religion was monodeism[3] (one god superior to all other gods who are inferior deities) as opposed to monotheism (one god, and a philosophical ethical system related to that god, with no other gods anywhere).

Another central concept of Judaism[B] was that man is by nature neither good nor evil, but both. These human qualities give man the freedom to choose between right and wrong. The choice belongs to man, not God.

In the entire Jewish tradition there is hardly any contempt shown for the human body, which rather is viewed as an essential instrument of life. Since God is not corporeal, and man sanctifies his own life because he is made in God's image, he must follow God's ways as he functions on earth. By sanctifying his own life and that of others, mankind is expressing love and honor for God. The sanctification of life is the primary theme of the Jewish religion. Since man by his free will can interfere with the course that God has set in motion, history can be seen as man acting for good or evil and receiving the appropriate consequence. When mankind finally lives a fit spiritual religious life and helps others to live this way, all of mankind will come to lead a godly life; then the messianic era will have arrived and not only will there be paradise in heaven but here on earth as well.

We can see that the basic concept of Judaism was love of all mankind. Love was continuously praised in the Old Testament: "to walk in all his ways, to love him, to serve the Lord your God with all your heart and all your soul"—"Love thy neighbor as thyself" (Deuteronomy 10.19-20; Leviticus 19.17).*

This theme of love prevailed in the family life of the Hebrews as well. And as you will see throughout the history of these people it distinguished them from their neighbors of the Middle East and Mediterranean basin.

In other ancient lands the abuse of woman and children, and even infanticide, was common. On, King of the Swedes,

---

* All biblical references are from the Old Testament, Masoretic text.

slew nine of his ten sons in the belief that he would prolong his life. The goddess Artemis was offended by the Greeks and required King Agamemnon to sacrifice his daughter Iphigenia. The Hebrews were willing to sacrifice everything (*akedah*) for the love of God, but were not required to make any actual human sacrifice because their God loved man and did not wish him any injury.

In looking at the fabric of the social structure, religious dicta, and history of the Hebrews, certain points stand out. "I have put before you life and death, blessings and curses, choose life" (Deuteronomy). This phrase "choose life" has become the central phrase for the Jewish attitude toward all of human life, as we will see by examining the history of these people.

The history of the Hebrews begins with Abraham, who came with his family from the ancient city of Ur on the Euphrates River in Sumeria, in approximately 2200 B.C., and settled in what would later become Palestine. These early Hebrews, known as Habiru, were a group of loosely united clans who wandered on the edge of the Arabian Desert. Borderline nomads, they were typical of a patriarchal family constellation. They were fighters and herdsman whose captives were used as servants. Because they were seminomadic, capturing large numbers of slaves was impractical for them. The children of the few slave captives they did have became hereditary property of the clan.

The Habiru kept sheep and goats, and when first noted in history they were settling in semipermanent communities. They viewed the desert as a refuge for outlaws and the home of demons and wild beasts. They rejected the sedentary life-style of civilizations of the cities, viewing them as morally and religiously perverse. They were borderland nomads, that is, they had simple community centers and herded their flocks in prescribed family/clan areas.

The Israelites, though broadly considered a patriarchy, were often fratriarchal: the eldest brother was head of the family, and passed on the rule to his eldest son. In addition, there were elements of an earlier matriarchy wherein the mother exercised authority and the child's lineage was traced through her, not through the father.

There is a close historical connection between the Hebrews and the Egyptians. During Egypt's Middle Kingdom (2500-1587 B.C.) the Hyksos—chiefs of nomadic tribes—and their partners, the Habiru, repeatedly invaded Egypt and finally controlled it until they were expelled by the founder of the 18th dynasty in 1587 B.C. The Hyksos and Habiru were considered barbaric by the Egyptians, but during their reign they did not destroy the religious or architectural wonders of the country and actually tried to develop what was there. Still, they were imprisoned and became slaves in this great period of construction. Egyptian history is sketchy here, but unlike other cultures of that time, the Hebrews wrote about their defeats and mistakes, as well as their victories, so our view is well-rounded.

The story of the Habiru exodus from Egypt is a tale of oppression under pharaoh Ramses II. The Hebrews who fled Egypt were led by Moses and Aaron and were an amalgamation of the Habiru slaves, Habiru who had intermarried with Egyptians, as well as Egyptians who fled along with them. They traveled for about 40 years, through two generations which eventually formed a new people—a series of tribes bound together loosely, led by Joshua. Together they crossed the Jordan and entered Canaan, occupying the land known as Palestine.

When Joshua died, there was anarchy, "where every man did what was right in his own eyes" (Judges 17.6). There was also a regression to the religious practices of neighbors, particularly the fertility rites that were rampant in Canaan at that time. We can safely assume that these Hebrews practiced infanticide and child sacrifices to foreign gods. This period precedes the biblical period of the Judges, when the last judge, Samuel, responded to the entreaties of the people who demanded that a king be selected, not to lead them in battle, but to judge them

(1 Samuel 8.5). Since Samuel feared that a king might become a tyrant, he required that there be a constitution to limit royal rights and powers (the first Magna Carta). In about 1025 B.C. Saul (1 Samuel 10.25) became the first constitutional monarch in the history of the world.

A golden era for Israel began with King David (1012-972 B.C.), who established a capital at Jerusalem and a sanctuary to house the Ark of the Covenant. He glorified the worship of Yahweh and established a religious liturgy. This era of growth soon began to crumble under the leadership of David's son, Solomon (971-931 B.C.), who did not discourage the pagan ideas of Israel's prosperous neighbors.

Solomon's death in 931 B.C. was followed by civil war and a resulting division of the land—Judah in the south, and a mightier, but heathenistic Israel to the north.

In 738 B.C. the armies of Tiglath-Pileser II conquered Israel, which had become disorganized, and was absorbed into Assyria. Judah, meanwhile, with only two tribes, remained as a nation, its religious precepts and laws intact. During this period the education of the people increased under the guidance of Jehoshaphat, whose goal was to spread the knowledge of the Book of the Lord to all the cities of Judah and to the world (2 Chronicles 17.9).

Some elements of idol worship crept into Judah and some Judean kings used murder as an instrument to extend their reigns. They also acknowledged the suzerainty of the Assyrians over Judah, thus allowing aspects of the Assyrian religion to be brought into their land. And so we find that child sacrifice was reinstituted. Sons were cast to the devouring fires of Moloch, a tyrant god of the ancient Phoenicians and Ammonites.

Around 640 B.C. Josiah instituted public education and public reading of the Torah. He also entered into a public covenant with the people and with God to end all public displays of idolatry. Still, despite his efforts idolatry was practiced in some private homes, due in part to the influence of corrupt priests who had lucrative practices in making animal sacrifices.

Judah was finally conquered during the Babylonian conquest, which began in 597 B.C. Its independence was lost, and its people were sent into permanent exile (the first Diaspora). This misfortune turned out to be a great educational experience for the people of Judah—who became known as Jews—and allowed them to develop a nation that remained intact for almost 25 centuries because of its culture, religion, and philosophy.

The Hebrews viewed themselves as having an intimate relationship with God, with whom they had three covenants. The first covenant was between Noah and God and was based on a belief in the sanctity of human life. Since blood was a symbol of life, God forbade the drinking of animal blood and required the penalty of death for any willful shedding of blood (Genesis 6.11). The second covenant was between God and Abraham through which God claimed Abraham and his descendants as his particular instruments. They were required to teach mankind "the way of the Lord to do righteousness and justice" (Genesis 18.19). The third covenant was made with all the Hebrews and was given by God to Moses on Mt. Sinai. The covenant required ratification of the two previous covenants, as well a commitment to the Ten Commandments. "And ye shall be unto me a kingdom of priests and a holy nation" (Exodus 19.6). This meant that all the people of Israel were required to be holy and render to mankind all services as a holy nation.

The Decalogue (Ten Commandments) was a unique moral statement. Unlike the laws of other nations, it forbade the deification of nature or the making of graven images (idols). It required observation of the Sabbath, honoring of parents, respect for property and life and the maintenance of a strong regard for a woman's honor. Further, there was the requirement to avoid any word or thought that might be potentially inimical to one's fellow man. This kind of law was unique in the world.

As a result of these laws there was no distinction between moral, religious, and secular laws. The religion and its laws were designed to transform the individual, his family, and society into a holy organization with service to others as the center of its system. It not only forbade idolatry, but also human sacrifice, prostitution (including sacred temple prostitution), divination, and magic. Thus, every social offense was a religious offense, and every religious offense a social offense against the fabric of the nation.

For the first time justice recognized six basic human rights: life, work, possessions, garments, shelter, and one's own person (which included leisure, liberty, and comfort). Further, there were direct prohibitions against hatred, vengeance, or carrying a grudge. Righteousness was a requirement of all the people, as well as concern for the poor, the weak, and the helpless, whether friend or foe.

The law did not see that the possession of earthly goods was a natural right, but a trust given by God to be respected and passed on to the next generation. The law directed the people to help a troubled neighbor and to avoid profiting from another's difficulty. "Thou shalt love thy fellow as thyself" (Leviticus 19.18). This righteousness was to include the non-Israelite stranger who lived among them, as well as humane treatment of all animals.

With an understanding of this unique moral code as a framework, let us now look at how the ancient Hebrews fared as a social structure, especially with regard to their treatment of women and children.

Marriage and home[4-10] were considered of fundamental importance to the ancient male Hebrew. Unless he had a wife, his home was not considered holy. And the home was the central institution in Judaism. At home the ideals of life were taught and developed. The home was sanctified and the marriage was the tie that made it so.

The Hebrew marriage was a sacred institution. Marriage was regarded as fundamentally holy because it was meant to produce two individuals who were in the image and likeness of God. "As soon as a man takes a wife his sins are buried; for it is said: who so takes a wife finds a great good and obtaineth favor from the Lord" (Talmud, Tractate Yebamoth, 63a-b). "When un-married a man diminishes the Divine image, for it is stated, in the image of God made ye man" (Midrash Rabbah Ecclesiastes 238-239).

With marriage came responsibility. A man was expected to care for his wife. It is stated repeatedly in Hebrew literature that it is a husband's duty to put his wife's care before his own. "It is better that I should go naked than not clothe my wife decently" (Jerusalem Talmud, Kethuboth, chapter 6,5). A dutiful husband should not aggravate his wife or cause her to shed tears. He should not be stingy in domestic expenses. Further, he was expected to love his wife like himself and respect her more than himself. According to the Talmud, a man was expected to do whatever his wife wished, so that his children would be rich in the love of their mother (Talmud, Bmutza, 59a; Yebamoth, 62b; Sanhedrin, 76a).

This prevailing attitude—to take care of and love one's wife so that she will care for and love one's children—is, I believe, fundamental in determining why child abuse and infanticide were rare among the ancient Hebrews. We will find later in our study that women who are abused are more likely to abuse their own children.

The Hebrew's attitude toward women and children[11-17]—particularly female children—was particularly protective for an-cient times.

When a daughter was born into a family she was cherished in a different way than a son. The moral responsibility of a father to his daughter was greater than to his sons "to prevent their degradation" (Talmud, Tractate Kethuboth, 49a). A father had certain rights over his minor daughter—rights not shared by a mother. To protect his daughter he could oversee betrothal. On the other hand, he had rights to the daughter's earnings from sewing or other handiwork; and he had the right to annul vows she had made. In the earliest Jewish history a father could even sell his daughter into servitude, though this later was prohibited. However, even in the earliest times when the daughter reached puberty these fatherly powers were completely lost. A female minor, though completely dependent upon her father for support, when reaching adolescence, could do as she wished. The minor child was more fully protected in Talmudic times[18-21] than before, since it became immoral to take away any article that the minor found or earned by dint of his or her efforts.

Upon the death of the father his heirs (the daughter's brothers) were required to give her a dowry based on the size of the father's estate had he lived. Her rights to her dowry came before the rights of the other heirs, and had to equal at least one-tenth of the estate. Any rights the daughter had from the mother's ketubah or marriage contract could not be withheld from her. Even if her mother waived this right it could not be removed. In pre-Talmudic times there was a primitive money, known as *mohar*, which was given to the father by the bridegroom to replace the loss of his daughter. Later this tradition was reversed. Fathers gave dowries instead to aid the young couple in their new life.

Though it was rare for a girl to take the initiative in courtship it did occur, and young people had ample opportunity to communicate and relate to each other. The young girls were not secluded. They were not veiled and it was acceptable for them to be with men in public.

During the Talmudic period the bridegroom provided a document to safeguard the bride's marital security (*kethubah*—a marriage contract). The *kethubah* would be read aloud, including the clause in which the bridegroom would pledge: "I will work for thee, I will honor thee, I will support and maintain thee, as it is seemly as a Jewish husband to do." Through the *kethubah* the bridegroom also declared how much he would give his bride if he ever divorced her or left her. The larger the amount, the more binding the pledge to remain with the woman.

Though polygamy was not forbidden by the Bible or even under Talmudic law, the ancient Hebrews generally disapproved of it and it was practiced by only very wealthy men and by kings during the monarchical period. Polygamy was officially outlawed by the 11th century B.C.

In the earliest part of their history the Hebrews had large families, patriarchies in which each family member was responsible for the other, and the head of the family was responsible for all. This biblical family was like a small religious community.

In biblical times, the children, particularly the sons, were extraordinarily important. Yet with all the importance of the patriarchal father, and the sons, who were the center of the many religious activities at home and in the community, the mother played a significant role in the family as well. Thus, it can be said that in biblical times there was a patriarchy in law and a matriarchy in family organization.

Rabbi Jacob said, "He who has no wife lives without good, or help, or joy, or blessing, or atonement." According to Rabbi Helbo, "Be careful about the honor of your wife, for blessing enters the house only because of the wife." Rabbi Elezar said, "If a man divorces his first wife, even the very altar sheds tears because of him." In the words of Rabbi Aha, "If a man marries a godly wife, it is as though he had fulfilled the whole Torah from beginning to end" (Talmud).

There were historically more rights and provisions given to Hebrew women than to women in the surrounding nations. Hebrew women were not truly equal under the law, but they were given equality in certain areas, and were stressed as superior in others. The Bible also records many female heroines: Miriam and Hulda, who were prophets, the judge Deborah, the exemplary mother Hannah, and the pious proselyte Ruth.

The sages believed that women were endowed with a greater understanding and intelligence (*binah*) than men. Further, women had the responsibility to run the home and raise the children and could not have two areas of responsibility—Torah study and the home. Thus, women were exempt, but not banned, from studying the Torah.

In the domestic world women were equal and in many

ways superior in their responsibilities. In the public world although women were exempt from public prayer, both men and women were required to read the Book of Esther. Some women became so knowledgeable about the Torah that they were able to add their wisdom to the Talmud (Beruriah, wife of Rabbi Meir). In penal and civil law women and men had equal status, and by Talmudic times women had a basic knowledge of the Bible and of the Talmud. In fact, it was considered valuable for a man to marry the daughter of a great scholar, as she was likely to be learned herself and could teach him. So we find that the wives of great scholars were treated with almost the same respect as their husbands. The Jews considered marriage and the sexual relation of husband and wife necessary for a religious home; while the Christians considered the sexual relations of husband and wife but a "necessary evil" to procreate. This was similar to the ancient Greek attitude.

The Bible instructs that fathers and mothers are both responsible for their children's care though they were each given very specific roles. We see the father's role as a protective warrior to be an extension of this maternalization process. A mother's role was different. She commanded automatic respect and obedience and was the central figure of love and unity within the family.

The central significance of a Jewish marriage[22-24] was the production of children, not only for family continuity, but as part of a divine role that was assigned to Israel. Parents were morally required to instruct their children in the practice and knowledge of Judaism, therefore children were vital for the continuity and dissemination of God's law.

If a mother refused to suckle her weakened child, the mother was considered worse than a monster (Job 39.14-16). However, if she was unable to suckle her baby, a wet nurse would be employed and the mother would be treated with every deference and consideration (Exodus 2.7-9). To illustrate the value placed upon mother and child, it is interesting to note that a lactating woman was given special privileges. A pregnancy could even be terminated if a women was lactating. The suckling mother could forgo religious requirements, profane the Sabbath, and eat nonkosher food, if it was deemed appropriate for her needs. The child's care came first (Talmud-Sabbath 129).

Children were weaned between 18 months and three years of age. This was an occasion to celebrate the passing of the dangerous age of infancy. From then on they were fed goat's milk. The milk of asses and camels was prohibited (this is interesting in that tuberculosis is not found in goats, but can be found in camels and asses). During the day the child would sleep in a cradle, but at night slept with its mother. There is some hidden evidence of maternal infanticide in that there were warnings about "overlaying the child by accident" (1 Kings 3.19). Still, in general, the Jewish mother was very nurturing of her children, as compared to mothers of some of the other cultures at that time.

Circumcision of the male infants was a widespread practice in the world. It was well known among the Egyptians (who did it when the child was older) as well as among the Mohammedans of more recent times. Only the Jews ritually circumcised on the eighth day after birth since the discomfort to the individual was considerably less, both physically and psychologically. At the time of circumcision the boys were named. Girls were named when the father was first called to read the Torah after her birth. The father redeemed the son at the time of circumcision (*pidyon-ha-ben*). Since in biblical times it had been required to be given to the priests to be taught and raised in the priesthood, the father had to symbolically purchase his son back from the priesthood with the promise that he would give him a proper education, a trade, and a wife (Talmud, Tractate Kiddush, 29a). Upon turning 13, when a Jewish boy reached his legal majority, the boy became a son of the covenant (bar mitzvah).

The Talmud has many rules about the proper treatment of children[25-29] and infants as well. It maintains that a baby should be bathed in warm water and rubbed with oil following the bath. (Hebrew children were considered so handsome by the Romans that during the Roman captivity they would tie Hebrew children to their beds when they had intercourse so that they might have handsome children as a result.)

As soon as a child was able to sit up, it would be dressed in a leather pinafore to "guard against the scratches by a cat" (Talmud). No child was to be left alone in its cradle by day or night, and it was fanned frequently to keep away the flies (Talmud, Chulin, 91b). "A baby should be as well looked after as is a king, high priest, and learned man" (Talmud, Yallinek Beth Hamidrash, Chapter 2, 96). During the biblical period, when a child was born, a cedar tree was planted for a boy and a pine tree for a girl to be used as poles for the *chuppah* (marriage canopy) when the child married.

Both mother and father had specific parental roles. For example, there were general social requirements for how a father was to educate and treat his children. The courts would penalize a father who shirked his duty. The courts were freer to deal with the wealthy man because they could force him to give *tzedakah* (charity/money) which would be turned over to his children and would be under the court's control.

The law[30,31] said that though the child was formed within the mother it was the father who was responsible for the way it developed. Until age six, both boys and girls were under the care and protection of the mother. Children received most of their early childhood religious education from their mothers. But at age six the boys only were placed directly under the father's control, education and instruction. According to the Talmud, this was a right of the child—to be cared for and to be instructed by the parent.

The male child was free of any legal or religious obligations until he was 13 years and one day old. He could not be punished for misdeeds until that age. The same was true of a female up until the age of 12. However, all children were expected to learn the practices of Judaism as they approached maturity.

As we can see, there was a strong intertwining of *father and son* and *teacher and pupil* among the ancient Hebrews. The father was admonished never to envy his son or pupil, nor favor one child over another. This relationship is characterized by a well known Talmudic statement. One of the three categories of people who will inherit the world to come are those who raise their children in the way of the Torah. According to the Talmud, the stubborn and rebellious son could be put to death—though there is no record of that occurring. This law was meant as a warning that the responsibility for the child's errant behavior was placed on the parents. "One should not promise a child to get him something and then not give it to him, because you will thereby teach him lying, as it is said, they have taught their tongues to speak lies" (Talmud).

We can see that the Jewish religion guided a child's development from the moment he was born. At birth the child was named and went through various religious rituals during its development, with increasing religious duties. During the entire period of a child's growth it was an intrinsic member of the family unit—literally from the day it was born. At age three a child was called a *katan*. The *katan* belonged to its father, so any legal contract signed by a *katan* also required the father as witness. He could contract marriage for his *katana* (daughter)[32], but at her majority she could refuse the marriage if she wished. A *katan* could be punished for having illegal intercourse; a *katana* could not. It was not considered a possibility for a girl to be sexually aggressive, e.g., to rape. Also, women were considered moral on a genetic basis—just because they were women.

From a girl's 12th birthday for six months and a boy's 13th birthday for six months, children were considered *na'ar* and their vows would be valid, but they had to be checked by a responsible adult. If there was no external evidence of puberty, that person was still considered a *katan* until age 20. If at 20 there was no evidence of puberty, then the person was considered impotent but was given adult status (Talmud).

In ancient Hebrew law there was no discrimination against bastard children, if the identity of the father was established. A father was obligated to insure his bastard child's daily care, to educate his son or daughter, and to teach the Torah and a profession to his sons, legitimate or not. There was no requirement to educate girls though such a girl would be more highly prized as a wife.

As we move from the early biblical period through the monarchies into the Talmudic and rabbinical period, we find that the relationship between father and children changes, with more love between parent and child and a less punitive attitude toward the child. Prior to this change there was always love bonding parent and child, typifying the relationship between God and His people. The early Bible threatened children with punishment for the sins of their parents. During the rabbinical period this situation was reversed, so that if a child suffered it was evident his parents had sinned. This is a marked social advance.

Among the ancient Hebrews, children were considered an important "bond of union between husband and wife" (Talmud). The male child was able to recite prayers in a synagogue after the parents died (*kaddish*), thus, occasionally a boy would be called a "*kaddish* for his parents." It is written in the Talmud that "Whoever leaves a son after him studying the Torah is considered as if he never died" and that sons and daughters of each marriage should be the result of true affection, for "he who marries for money shall have worthless children."

The age of the child (boys in very early times and both boys and girls by Talmudic times) and his mental abilities would determine what rights he had to his own property and the results of his labor. By the time he reached maturity he could fulfill all legal obligations. There was only one limitation: the land and property of a deceased father could not be sold until the male child was 20 years old (Talmud Tractate Gittin, 64b, 65a).

Though the father had extensive rights over his children, he was prohibited from giving corporal punishment to his grown children (Talmud, Moed Katon, 17a); and where the Bible speaks of the rights of the father to sell his daughter to be a maidservant it is primarily in the oldest part of the Bible and does not include the postbiblical period when there were more restrictions.

A parent's responsibility for children included providing an education of the development of sexuality. Male masturbation was disapproved. It was considered such an abomination that the Talmud required that the genitals not be touched during urination. For boys, touching any part of the body below the umbilicus was discouraged (Talmud, Niddah, 13a). This was not the case with girls. The Talmud did not impose such restrictions upon them because it was believed that girls were not so easily excited. In fact, girls were advised to examine their genitals with a swab regularly to see whether they were menstruating. "A man who willingly causes an erection shall be placed under the ban. But why did he not say, this is forbidden? Because the man really incites his evil inclination against himself. He is called a renegade, because such is the art of the evil inclination: today it incites man to do one wrong thing, and the next, incites him to worship idols, and he then proceeds to worship them." "Thou shalt not commit adultery" implies, thou shalt not practice masturbation either with hand or with foot. Further, the rabbis taught: Prostitutes and those that play with children delay the advent of the Messiah. Those that practice pederasty are such people who are subject to stoning. Those that practice onanism: are they not deserving of destruction by flood?" (Talmud, Tractate Niddah 88).

Sexuality during marriage[33,34] was considered normal, though premarital sex was to be avoided. Though the purpose of sexual relations was to have children, a man who could no longer have children was still urged to avoid the celibate life.

"An unmarried man is only half a body and becomes a complete human only when he marries" (The Sages).

A man was forbidden to compel his wife to have sexual relations. "Whosoever compels his wife to the marital obligation will have unworthy children. What is the scriptural proof? Also without consent the soul is not good" (Rabbi Joshua Ben Levi). "A woman who solicits her husband to the marital obligation will have children the like of whom did not exist even in the generation of Moses" (Talmud, Tractate Erubin, 100b).

Traditional Hebrew law (*halakhah*) gave special rules for the *onah* (sexual relations between husband and wife). These laws required a man to satisfy his wife's sexual needs and forbade him from raping her. The rules required that a wife had merely to be inviting in her appearance and dress and to indicate in a nonverbal way that she had sexual needs. Her husband was required to meet them. The *halakhah*, in fact, was more permissive and generous to the woman than to the man. It granted all rights for the sexual satisfaction of the woman and placed great restraints on the man.

The Talmudic order "Do not profane thy daughter to cause her to be a whore" referred not only to a disdain for incest, but also warned against the arrangement of marrying a daughter off to an older man. Though it was permitted by early biblical law for a poor man to sell his daughter to another as a bondwoman, during the rabbinical period it was considered such a wretched act that rabbis warned against it. They said it was comparable to selling a Torah, which was considered the worst blasphemy.

According to Jewish law every other sexual relationship outside of marriage was considered deviant. Though sexual relations between unmarried people or lesbians were restricted, they were not considered transgressions (Leviticus 18). Adultery was most strenuously condemned. Though a married woman was forbidden to have sexual relations with any man except her husband, a married man was free to have sexual relations with any other woman, as long as she was single and available, which indicates the inequality between the sexes.

In the early biblical period adultery was punished by death. During the Talmudic period this evolved into a more benign response. The Talmud provided a test to determine whether a woman was guilty of adultery—the "test of the bitter water." A special solution was mixed of water, dust from the temple grounds, and ink with which curses had been written on a scroll. If the accused woman could drink this water with no ill effects she was considered innocent. Of course this test practically guaranteed that any woman who declared herself innocent would be innocent. If a woman was found guilty of adultery she would be divorced by her husband and could not marry her lover.

An unmarried, unbetrothed woman[35,36] was permitted to have sexual relations. If a single woman had an exclusive sexual relationship with a man whom she could legally marry (if they had wished), their relationship was considered a common-law marriage. If she transferred her alliance to another man without first obtaining a divorce (*get*) from the first, she could be considered an adulteress, for which she would be punished. The commentaries in the Talmud condemn these nonmarital sexual experiences as promiscuous, though not adulterous. (Sexual relations of a married woman with someone other than her husband was adultery. Sexual relations of a single woman was not called adultery.)

Lesbianism was not considered a true sexual deviance, and was not even mentioned in the Bible. In fact, it was never considered a possibility. In later Talmudic writings, when it was understood that sexual acts could occur between women, it was never explicitly prohibited as a sexual transgression, since there was no actual genital union. It was a man's responsibility to supervise his wife and provide her with sexual fulfillment so that she would not feel the need of these deviant relationships.

The homosexuality referred to in Leviticus 18 and 20 as an abhorrence was strictly between men.

Jewish literature held high moral standards for Jews and criticized non-Jews (particularly the Hellenes) for their proclivity for homosexuality and other "heathen indulgences," including bestiality. In Leviticus 18 we read that sexual transgressions were such that the very land where they were committed became so defiled that the Jews had to leave Sodom.

War was common in the biblical period. Since Jews were sometimes taken captive in lands with loose moral codes, the rabbis feared that a captured girl could lose her virginity and become ineligible for marriage. They ruled that any minor younger than 3 years and a day could not lose her virginity no matter what was done to her. If she were older she could have her virginity exposed (lost) and still be given as a bride. The final arrangements of actually living together would not take place until many years later when she reached her sexual majority. At that point the young woman could accede to or refuse the marriage. The logic of this arrangement was actually a loophole in Jewish law. If a girl was ransomed and returned from captivity, she would either be considered a virgin (if she were under three) or an engaged woman who had been violated by a stranger and was thereby still acceptable as a bride (Talmud, Ketuboth, 1:2).

As we see, the ancient Hebrews took a curious view of the sexuality of man as compared to woman. They discouraged women from participating in public readings of the Torah because they were concerned that a man seeing a woman might have sexual thoughts and would be distracted from his study. It was not considered that a woman could be distracted by the men.

Women were exempt from the commandment to procreate. Procreation was a man's responsibility, thus allowing women the right to use contraception. A woman could obtain a divorce (*get*) from her husband if he refused to procreate. However, a man could not force his wife to use contraception against her will. The Talmud has many references to how women should use contraceptive devices and exercise their freedom to avoid pregnancy. As you may imagine, this was an unusual legal prerogative in the ancient world, particularly in a society that had so stressed procreation and family life. The rabbis reasoned that if a woman had an unwanted pregnancy she might be a poorer mother and might injure that child or an older child she was caring for.

The primary contraceptive device was a *mokh*. It was a very fine soft cotton on which was placed a chemical organic material. It was used as a tampon to block the cervix as well as a spermicide. The Talmud even indicated that minors, pregnant women, and nursing mothers could and should use the *mokh*, because a minor might become pregnant and die, a pregnant woman might cause injury to the fetus, and a nursing woman might have to wean her child prematurely (Yebamot 12b).

The *halakah* permitted abortion when it was necessary to save the mother's life (Ocholot 7:6). In fact, if a pregnant woman were sentenced to death, an abortion would precede the penalty unless she was near term. This procedure upheld the law, for if the woman had to wait to deliver the child, she would be psychologically tormented and torture was not permitted by the Talmud. If she were pregnant from a rape, the pregnancy could be aborted, unless the pregnancy were near term. And to qualify as near term, a hand or a finger had to show from the birth canal. The *halakah* viewed rape as intercourse forced upon a woman, even by a husband. If the primary motivation for sexual activity was violence, not sexual gratification, that was also considered rape (Baba Kama 63b). If a rape began under duress but the woman became a more willing participant and continued the sexual activity, it was still classified as a rape.

As in many other ancient cultures menstruation was considered an unclean state. The Talmud instructed a man to avoid his wife for seven days because while in contact with her he might develop an aversion for her; this precaution was "so that she shall be beloved by her husband as at the time of her first entry into the bridal chamber" (Talmud, Tractate Niddah, 31b). Though a woman was considered unclean she was not considered unacceptable because she was menstruating. We must remember that during ancient and unsophisticated times the sight of blood frightened people, because it was usually a sign of illness. Illness was not only feared, but like a menstruating woman it was to be avoided. Yet, they believed that it was good for a woman to have regular menstrual periods. Some of these disparaging attitudes have remained over time. Still, Rabbi Hiyya taught that "as leaven is wholesome for the dough so is menstrual blood wholesome for a woman." And according to the Talmud: "Every woman who has an abundance of menstrual blood has many children" (Talmud, Tractate Niddah, 64lb).

During *niddah* (the menstrual period), the woman was not socially or religiously ostracized, though she usually did avoid the synagogue. The origin of the word *niddah* referred to being ostracized or excluded, indicating that the menstrual material makes the woman unacceptable. This concept changed over time. In the early biblical period a woman was ostracized. In the Talmudic period she was partially unclean. Later, *niddah* was only significant in laws of coitus with the husband.

Though it is true that *niddah* separated men from women, it is worth noting that both the Talmud and the Bible emphasize the equality of responsibility of mother and father in the moral and ethical sphere of training the child. It is also noteworthy that four mothers, or matriarchs in the Bible (Sarah, Rebecca, Rachel, and Leah) are ranked equally with the three patriarchs (Abraham, Isaac, and Jacob).

The laws of courtship and betrothal had developed to such an extent that by 200 A.D. all marriages were preceded by an engagement and a marriage contract, and no intercourse was permitted until after the wedding ceremony. Punishment for breaking these rules was severe: 40 lashes to the man who incorrectly obtained a wife. The Talmud stated, "and whoever lives without a wife lives without well being, without blessing, without a home, without Torah, without protective wall, without peace." Thus, the Hebrews were required to be married, enjoy companionship, and then procreate in order to perpetuate the pact between God and Israel.

Wife-beating was considered more serious than assaulting another man, because it was a violation of the duty to honor one's wife. The punishment for the man was very severe. If a husband and wife both accused each other in front of the courts, the husband's testimony was discounted. Women were considered generally law-abiding and more truthful.

"The heart of her husband does safely trust in her and he has no lack of gain. She does him good and not evil all the days of her life. Strength and dignity are her clothing; and she laughs at a time to come. She opens her mouth with wisdom; and the law of kindness is on her tongue. She looks well to the ways of her household and eats not the bread of idleness. Her children rise up and call her blessed; her husband also comments and he praises her: many daughters have done valiantly, but you exceed them all. Grace is deceitful and beauty is vain; but a woman that fears the Lord, she shall be praised. Give of the fruit of her hands; and let her works praise her in the gates" (Proverbs 31.10-31).

As their intricately and thoroughly codified life-style matured, the ancient Hebrews refined their laws and moral standards. Keep in mind that there remained an order in the relationship between the philosophy, culture, religion, and law of the Jewish people. For example, it was believed that the most dangerous vices were envy, greed, and pride (Ethics of the Fathers 4.2). Though asceticism was antithetical and alien to the spirit of Judaism, self-control was considered a moral attribute. Therefore, the body was not viewed as a contaminated vessel or its appetites evil (as by many other religious and cultural groups). One could not neglect one's body and its physical needs whether it related to food, rest, or sex. All were meant to glorify God.

The laws that ruled the Hebrews matured as well. In pre-Diaspora Hebraic law, for example, the following punishments prevailed:

1. Death by stoning, burning, decapitation, or strangulation.
2. Excision.
3. Death at the hands of heaven.
4. Banishment.
5. Corporal punishment (flogging).
6. Monetary fines.
7. Servitude.
8. Imprisonment.
9. Excommunication.
10. Death at the hand of a zealot.

In the Bible, capital punishment as a threat was considered a deterrent. "All Israel shall hear and fear and shall do no more any such wickedness in the midst of thee" (Deuteronomy 13.12). Murder was a crime against the sanctity of the land and no expiation could be made. Therefore, capital punishment ceased to be inflicted by Hebrew courts since long before the destruction of the second temple. When, in ancient times, the death sentence was still utilized, it was for the crimes of idolatry, profaning the Sabbath, father's incest, rape of a betrothed girl, adultery, and murder.

The most common punishment was flogging, and this was administered by the court under the supervision of a physician who would determine how long the accused could endure the punishment. The physician could stop the flogging at any time.

Offenses against property were punishable by a fine, and personal injury only required financial restitution. When a man was unable to repay the value of the theft, he could be sold to

reading and writing at home by their mothers so they could teach their young children.

By the second Diaspora the Hebrews became multi-lingual.[44-47] They spoke Aramaic in their homes and learned Greek for business and culture. They learned Latin to deal with the Romans, in addition to Hebrew for scriptural study, and local languages as well.

According to the Talmud a father was required to teach his son whatever was necessary for him to survive in the world. For example, the father was expected to teach his son to swim because he could then help save the life of someone who might be drowning.

At age six, a boy, if he could pass the medical examination and was seen as physically fit to receive instruction, was sent to Talmudic school (Talmud, Baba Bathra, 21a; Kethuboth, 50a). Going to school was considered such a great honor that the mother would carefully wash and dress her child as a duty and privilege, and accompany him to school (Talmud, Berachoth, 17a).

To prevent the fatherless child from growing up ignorant, Joshua Gemala established schools in every small town and village with compulsory education for all boys above the age of six (Talmud, Sotah, 22a). In fact, a community could be compelled to build a school. "An empty-headed man cannot be a sin-fearing man, nor can an ignorant person be pious" (Hillel, 50 B.C.).

From postbiblical times there was always a minority that championed the cause of female education and even advocated equal rights for both male and female minors. In some schools (Palestine) daughters were taught but they generally received their training in the Scriptures only (Talmud, Nedashin, 4.3).

Beginning under the direction of Ezekiel, who was the first of a long line of scribes/teachers known as *soferim*, the Torah began to occupy a more central place in the life of the people. The first Diaspora ended in 538 B.C. with the fall of Babylon to Cyrus of Persia. But when the people were permitted to return to their land of Judah many stayed behind in the cities where they had established themselves not just in commerce but in education.

At this time a reorganization of the land of Israel took place with the reestablishment of Judea under Cyrus the Great. However, an inadequate number of teachers was available in Judea to teach the Torah. Though the center of the country was theoretically Judea, the main cultural and educational center for the Hebrews was still in Babylon. To assist the people of Judea to absorb and understand their history and religion, the learned Hebrews in Babylon began writing Torah commentaries which eventually became the Babylonian Talmud, making the Torah accessible to all.

Judaism began to change from a priestly religion to a religion that was concerned with all questions of life and human relationships. Since the Talmud was written in the vernacular it could be read and studied by all. A "state" thereby developed that had no boundaries: a state ruled by a book called the Torah. Thus began the first truly theocratic, legalistic, and moralistic state.

Because of the wide dispersion of the Hebrews in various lands, and because of language differences, the Hebrews began to use Greek as the lingua franca. They produced a Greek version of the Bible called the Septuagint (in memory of the 70 elders). This version (280 B.C.) was the oldest known version of the Bible until the discovery of the Dead Sea Scrolls. It was used to carry the message of Judaism to the entire world.

The Torah, along with the Babylonian Talmud[48] (and, today, with the Jerusalem Talmud[49]), the Midrash, and the Mishnah became the written[50-55] established authority that could travel anywhere in the world and be used as a repository for knowledge and information on how to live as a Torah Jew. I think of it as being the first traveling university—one that was transmitted around the world.

The Talmud was, and still is, a text of morality and history that covers all of religion and ethics; it is encyclopedic. It con-

tains reflections, homilies, apologias, maxims, wisdom, specula-
tions, stories, histories, and legends, as well as scientific observations about geometry, medicine, astronomy, botany, and
physiology. Its aim and purpose is to inspire, edify, and raise a
person to the highest qualities of their mind and heart, "to be
righteous in the name of the Lord."(56-59)

To make this "university" most effective, it was required
that all Hebrew males be literate in the Bible, which was in
Hebrew, and in the Talmudic material, which was in the vernacular Greek, Aramaic, etc. This made the Hebrews the first
people in the history of mankind whose male population was
100% literate. It also made them the first people who could
communicate across borders and empires with clarity. This unified the Hebrews in their philosophy and basic cultural structure.

We see that their study of religion was designed to be practical; it explained how to conduct one's daily life in relationship
to the will of God. Righteousness was the supreme law of the
world and the basic essential attribute of God. The Jews believed
that what was true and right in one place was true and right
everywhere; that man is a unity and any violation of that unity
was an injury to God and his righteousness. God was not only
seen as part of the moral order, but the entire order of living for
all mankind.

The sages (*hakamim*, biblical period, premonarchical),
along with the prophets and wise men, wrote the Book of Proverbs, Job, and Ecclesiastes. They appealed to reason and wisdom and proclaimed knowledge as vital for man's worth;
knowledge to be used not to help himself, but to help his down-
trodden neighbor. It was a literature full of wisdom and
compassion:

To know wisdom and instruction;
to comprehend the words of understanding;
to receive the discipline of wisdom,
justice, and to right inequity,
to give prudence to the simple,
to the young man knowledge and discretion. (Proverbs 1.2-4)

What is primarily different in the wisdom of the sages compared to that of the Canaanites, Egyptians, Babylonians, Medes, and Greeks is that there is a moral foundation directly related to God for the development of wisdom. The Hebrews believed that the development of wisdom is for the goal of righteousness, not just for the purpose of gaining knowledge.(60-62)

The Code of Hammurabi and the Code of the Hittites were created to protect property, while the Torah was for the protection of the person. For example, the Torah forbade the employer to exploit his workmen or even his slaves. Even the creditor was not allowed to affront the dignity of the person who was in debt to him (Leviticus 19.13; Deuteronomy 24.10-11).

The Torah also stated that a slave had the rights of a person. In fact, if he were physically injured by his owner, he was automatically freed (Exodus 21.26-27). Furthermore, if the slave ran away and was found by another man, the man who found the slave was forbidden to return him to his master (Deuteronomy 21.16-17). The Hammurabi Code required the death penalty for those who aided a runaway slave.

From their earliest history slavery was always a part of the Hebrew world, whether they were slaves themselves or owners. When Israel and Judah were divided, Israel had a large slave population. During the period of Herod (a non-Jew) there was extensive use of slaves in building projects for the glorification of Herod (and the Roman emperor), and to house troops. But, although it did exist, slavery among the Hebrew people was generally limited.

Even though there was slavery in the world and among the Hebrews, they considered freedom an inalienable right. In Job 31.13-15 we read, "If I despise the cause of my man servant or my maid servant, when they contend with me; what then shall I do when God rises up? And when He visiteth, what shall I answer him? Did not He that made me in the womb make him? And did not One fashion us in the womb?"

So it was forbidden to let a slave perform any work that was not absolutely necessary. Even a disabled slave had to be cared for with the same solicitude as one who was healthy. Most slaves of the Hebrews were used for agricultural labor and in domestic situations where they were considered part of the household and participated in all the family's religious activities. Since so many of the religious activities were centered in the home, slaves participated equally. During the biblical period there were many free dependents who participated in a similar manner and there was no clear distinction between them and the slaves in the home.

The Bible described the slave as more than a bondsman. The slave was never treated as a nonhuman. The Hebrew who became a slave did so in payment of a debt or voluntarily sold himself because of poverty. He had to be redeemed from slavery after six years of service or earlier if he paid the balance of his debt (Exodus 21.7-11; Leviticus 25.39). "Who so acquires a slave to himself acquires a master to himself" (Kiddush 20a).

A non-Hebrew slave or bondsman was regarded more as the property of his master and could be bequeathed to his heirs together with his other possessions. However, the ancient Hebrews could not mistreat the non-Hebrew slave. If abuse did occur the slave was automatically released. He was also released during the jubilee year, which occurred every 50 years.

The non-Hebrew slave was made part of the home. If the slave was male, he was circumcised and was considered part of the community. Not only was he allowed to but he was requested to participate in all the religious duties of the community and of the home in which he lived. Furthermore, if he made full conversion to Judaism, once he was accepted as a full Jew, he would be automatically released from slavery. False conversions were rare, as he had to convince a court of three rabbis of his sincerity. The female slave was a domestic servant. If she was used sexually, she automatically became a concubine, no longer a slave, and could request becoming a second wife. Not long after the second Diaspora (Roman), slavery disappeared among the Jews.

The rest of the world, primarily the Greeks and the Romans, laughed at the Hebrews for giving such freedom, care, and concern to their slaves, particularly for giving them the Sabbath as a day of rest. In these other countries the kidnapping of people for slavery was considered a reasonable commercial activity. If a Hebrew kidnapped someone this was classified as a capital crime. There were additional humanitarian laws that provided for a slave laborer to receive his wages at the end of every day.

It must be noted that female slaves had fewer rights than male slaves, and it was much more difficult for a female slave to obtain her freedom. One important exception was if she married a member of the household. This happened often, and resulted in her slave status being lifted. This concept was incomprehensible to the Greeks, who considered slaves nonhumans.

In biblical times an Israelite father could sell his daughter to be a slave/concubine to another man's son. She would not be freed in the seventh year like a male slave, but if her master was dissatisfied with her, he could sell her back to her family, but not to a stranger. If the master took another wife he was expected to leave the slave girl's rights intact. If he intended for the slave girl to be his son's wife, he had to treat her as a daughter and not as a slave. It is interesting to note that this law also applied to women who were captured by the Hebrews and were later married by their captors.

But these laws were part of early Hebrew history and were changed as the culture became more sophisticated. At a later date we find that the female Israelite slave had the same rights as the male Israelite slave and was freed in the seventh year unless she refused her freedom and chose to remain a member of the family.

Once a slave was freed he or she did not join an underclass in society. Upon liberation the former slave belonged once more to the people of the land. However, there were inequities. The large slave population—actually, prisoners of war—that worked the mines and foundries under King Solomon worked under terrible conditions. The rate of mortality must have been high. But this occurred only during the monarchical period. By the time of the Babylonian exile slavery completely disappeared.

Overview

Before the Hebrews were a true nation they were a small group of Semitic tribesmen with family continuity and typical patriarchal practices. Following the Exodus from Egypt, if not before, strict rules of conduct were established not only by their leaders but, they believed, as a command and requirement from God. Isolated from others in the desert, the ancient Hebrews formed a society of strong family cohesiveness, continuity with ancestors, and they did this—unlike the cultures that surrounded them—with a relative absence of abuse to their children.

For the Hebrews, there was only one God (also uncharacteristic in that God was noncorporeal). God gave man all the qualities of good and evil and endowed him with free will and the responsibility to choose between the two. Furthermore, God was for all mankind, not just for the Jews. This made the Hebrews part of humanity, not separate from it, and their main function was to communicate the word of God to the world.

Ancient biblical law required that all men be learned and that women understand the faith. As a result, women were only educated to a partial degree. The Hebrews soon became the most educated and literate culture the world had ever known. Earlier than for any other people, Hebrew law and custom required elementary instruction for all children in the community, rich and poor alike, male and, eventually, female.

This was a culture that through law and God's word revered and respected life and the living. It was a culture whose foundation was based among peoples whose life-styles were often inhumane, where men mistreated, maimed, and killed their women and children, and where torture was commonplace.

The Hebrews protected their women and children and protected the strong love and family-based culture their law and their God created. Tacitus, the great Roman historian who lived around 55 A.D., viewed the Hebrews as contemptible because "they considered it a crime among them to kill any child."

Thus the Hebrews, though similar to many other peoples, and derived from the cultures around them, developed their own unique and moral contribution to the civilization of man.

Chapter 5

Rome: The Power and Some Glory

Quod licit jovi . . . non licit bovi. (What is permitted Jove . . . is not permitted cows.)

Our language, our cities, our law, and perhaps even our way of family life can be viewed as a complicated continuation of those of the ancient world's greatest military giant—Rome. We have long anticipated our visit, hoping somehow to witness the splendors of early civilization at its best. The year is 82 A.D. The spectacular amphitheater, the Colosseum, has just been completed—an icon of Roman superiority—and we approach it with awe. As we walk under the high exterior arches and through the gates we see marble—seats supported by vaulted galleries arranged in tier after tier as if they were reaching for the Roman heavens.

The place is filled to capacity today with 45,000 raucous Romans, and apparently the show is about to begin. As it does, the magnificence that is Rome—her architectural beauty, her prosperous orchards, her luxurious life-style—is soiled by the horrifying spectacle that follows as the gladiators are mutilated to the cheers of the crowd.

The show today, and every day, is death—meaningless,

brutal, and often lustful—a grotesque juxtaposition to the surrounding beauty that was Rome.

The organization of the ancient cities of the Italian peninsula(A) was similar to that of Greece. The Etruscans controlled a series of independent city-states which united only occasionally against an external foe. All of the city-states fell into Roman hands after the 6th century B.C. The development of the Etruscan civilization and culture had been more advanced than that of the Romans; much of it taken from Assyria, Babylonia, Egypt, and Greece.

The original Romans were apparently from Villanova, north of the Tiber. They formed their first major city at Alba Longa, on the slopes of the Alban Hills. Rome was just another small village as late as the 7th century B.C. But because of its commanding location on the Tiber River it grew in size and prominence. By 560 B.C. the population of Rome had reached 260,000.

This all happened within the first major period of Roman history when Rome was a monarchy. This period lasted from 753 to 509 B.C. It was followed by the period of the Republic (509-27 B.C.), the Empire (27 B.C.-476 A.D.), and later, by medieval and modern Rome. King Servius Tullius, whose reign lasted approximately from 578 to 535 B.C., fortified the city and established a class system based on property. Within 100 years Rome was declared a Republic. The last Etruscan king, Tarquinius Superbus, was expelled and the first councils were established. Though Rome was now free, the Etruscans were still the most powerful people in the area and the Romans were subject to them. It is pertinent to note that the Etruscans were similar to the people of Crete (Minos) both genetically and culturally. Their barbaric origin made them particularly cruel and they typically sacrificed animals and people in their religious rituals. Many human victims were slaughtered, even buried alive, at the funerals of important Etruscan leaders. Sometimes numbers of their war prisoners would be massacred as an offering to the gods.

The Gauls attacked Rome in 390 B.C. While the Romans rebuilt the city and strengthened its walls, they also decided to rewrite their own history. They invented a series of myths about their origin in an attempt to build up their national self-esteem.

In 451 B.C. Roman senators went to Athens to study the laws of Solon in order to establish a Roman legal system based on Solon's Grecian model. By the end of the 4th century the Romans defeated the Gauls, who had settled in Northern Italy in 350 B.C. At this time, the Romans began building the Appian Way. It was a period of extensive development in Rome. In fact, the Romans adopted their well known arched ceilings from Etruscan architecture (which was originally based on the Egyptian arch).

One way to examine Rome is by surveying its military movements. In 222 B.C. the Romans conquered Northern Italy where they met and fought with the Carthaginians. By the end of the third Punic war in 146 B.C. Roman forces had destroyed Carthage and massacred 450,000 of its inhabitants. They sold the remaining 50,000 into slavery. Rome now consisted of Sicily, Sardinia, Corsica, all of the Italian Peninsula, Spain, Southern Gaul and the Transalpine area, as well as North Africa and Macedonia.

In 60 B.C. Caesar returned to Rome as the elected Consul and formed the first Triumvirate with Pompey and Crassus. Twelve years later Caesar succeeded against Pompey and became the first dictator, though he was assassinated one year later. Octavian, Caesar's adopted nephew, renamed himself Augustus and became the first true emperor of Rome. In 40 B.C. Herod (mentioned in Chapter 4) was appointed King of Judea. From 164 to 180 A.D., during the reign of Marcus Aurelius, a plague ravaged the Roman Empire, limiting its expansionist thrust and encouraging better government management. By 200 A.D. Carthage, a Roman city, was again a major world metropolis, and by 212 A.D. Roman citizenship was given to every freeborn subject in the Empire. The "barbarians" (Visigoth, Goth,

Ostrogoth, and others) successfully invaded all parts of the Empire and repeatedly had to be driven out. Diocletian (284-305 A.D.) divided the Empire into east and west and in 337 A.D. Emperor Constantine reunited it. By 340 A.D. the Empire was again divided into east and west—a move from which it never truly recovered. By 476 A.D. the Western Roman Empire was ending and all that remained of the Empire in the East was Constantinople, its capital.

That is a capsulized version of the story of ancient Rome, which tells us very little of what actually took place within the Roman Empire—about family life and the sociological developments that took place over the years.

Magic, witchcraft, demonology, and the wish to manipulate the invisible powers of the gods were important aspects of life in this ancient world.[1-3] All classes of citizens, even the most sophisticated, believed that dangerous supernatural powers operated and controlled their lives. In fact, all the ancient civilizations believed in magic. They believed that the positions of the planets, the signs of the zodiac, and their relationship to each other governed the destiny of human beings. The roots of this magical thinking are prehistoric, and probably can be traced back to some cult of an earth goddess (fertility) or to the ancients' awe of the power of the sun.

The Jews were considered formidable magicians by the Romans[4] and the various names of their deity were used in many Roman magical papyri. Evidence of this was found buried in Alexandria and other sites, inscribed with the names Jao (Yahweh) Sabaoth, and Adonai. That the Jewish God could not be seen made him even more magically powerful.

In antiquity, mediums were often used to communicate with the other world and so-called "natural" mediums were found among young boys. Adults would try to get young boys to go into trances so that they could contact and communicate with dead ancestors.

Belief in demons and demonology was extensive and crucial to certain religious activities. For centuries the early Roman Christians believed in the reality and power of pagan gods—not considered as powerful as God the Father and the Son. These pagan gods had to be reckoned with as evil spirits and as demons. Along with this ideology came the concept of exorcism. The patrician would not leave his house without consulting the gods; until he had completed an expiatory ceremony, he would tremble in fear of their possible wrath. In general one can say that the Romans were suspicious, distrustful, cruel, highly superstitious, and fearful of offending any god anywhere.

The foundations of the home of Julius Caesar Germanicus contained human remains and magical curse tablets engraved with his name. Curse tablets were used extensively. Their magic is explained and incantations are found in a number of papyri now preserved in European museums. The most powerful in the land not only believed in magic, but that human sacrifice could make them more powerful.

Romans believed that after death people continued to live underground with the same human frailties they had when they were alive. Even underground they needed food and water. Therefore, on certain days of the year a meal was carried to the tomb, and surrounded by wreaths of grass, flowers, cakes, fruits, milk, and wine, and sometimes even blood, which was considered the vital life force. According to Cicero: "Our ancestors desire that the men who well acquitted this life should be counted in the number of the gods."

In the house of every Roman an altar held a small quantity of ashes and a few lighted coals. It was the sacred obligation of the master of the house to maintain this fire at all times, for the Romans believed that if it were extinguished, the family would be extinguished as well. One day each year, on the first of March, each family snuffed its sacred fire and lit another immediately. The fire was divine and was adored as if it were a god. Religion ruled every aspect of the ancient Roman's daily life. Every act had rigid controls attached to it. Every meal was a religious act. When he left the house, he would meet sacred objects everywhere and have to pronounce an immediate prayer. Sometimes he would have to turn his head to avoid seeing an object that boded ill. He made private sacrifices at home every day, and every month he joined with others of his tribe to offer group sacrifices. He never left his house without looking to see if a bird or other ill omen would appear. There were words he would not pronounce his entire lifetime, since they were "evil." If he had some desire he would write his wish on a tablet and place it at the feet of a statue of a divinity. At every moment of his life he would consult the gods to know their wishes. He would never make a decision without the interpretation of the entrails of victims, or the flight of birds, or of lightning to learn the predictions. The ancient Romans did not have much liberty in their private lives, their education, or religion. The individual counted for little. Divine authority and the state counted for all.

Each family, then, had its own hearth,(5-8) its own fire, and its own god, which it did not share with other families. It was the son's duty to make libations and sacrifices to his father and his ancestors. Any failure to perform these duties was considered the grossest act of impiety, equal to an act of patricide, multiplied as many times as there were male ancestors. Death was the punishment.

When a father gave life to his son, or allowed him to live, he also gave him his creed and worship, the right to continue the sacred fire, to offer the funereal meal in honor of dead ancestors and to say the various prayers, to honor his father alive and when dead. This established a mysterious bond between father and son, which should not be viewed as affection. Historians of Roman law have remarked that neither birth nor love was the foundation of the Roman family. Rather, it was founded on religious rules and the power of the father and husband. This ancient family was united by something considered more powerful than birth, emotional attachment, or physical strength.

They were drawn together by the religion of the sacred fire and their worship of dead ancestors.

A wife gave up worship at her parents' home and joined in the worship of her new ancestors once she got married. She could not belong to two families at the same time, and she could only have one domestic religion.

The Roman religion (which changed later in the empire) stressed the unacceptability of celibacy—a grave impiety. Male children were needed to keep the religious fire lit and to worship dead ancestors. The son owed everything to his father and the father depended on his son.

Religion, not laws, also determined the rights to property. Every domain was under the control of household divinities. The family's real estate was surrounded by a special enclosure— an uncultivated band of soil several feet wide—which separated it from the domain of other families. It was a sacred space. On appointed days a religious ceremony was held on this ground and the father and his family would walk around the border carrying sacrificial victims. Land could never be given as an inheritance to a son, but was passed on to the next supervisor of the family fortune which went from generation to generation; it belonged in the family. The family was part of the land.

Just like the land, women and children[9-18] were also the property of the head of the household. For example, a daughter was under her father's control until he died, and then her brother became her master. When she married, she came under the guardianship of her husband. If her husband died, she remained under the guardianship of her husband's agnates, and even her own sons. In cases such as these, the son had the authority to designate a guardian for his mother or could even choose a second husband for her.

The derivation of the word *pater*, as in *paterfamilias*, gives us some idea of the actual role of the father in ancient Rome. It did not mean paternity. The word, from its Indo-European root, referred to authority and majestic dignity of an almost godlike quality. Thus, the *paterfamilias* was the supreme authority of the domestic religion. He could accept a child at its birth or choose to kill it. He could repudiate his wife if she were sterile. He could exclude a son from the family and family worship if he did not approve of his son's behavior—or, worse, he could sell him into slavery. If he wished, he could introduce a stranger to the domestic hearth by adopting him. The father's will was absolute.

A father could be governed by the state for acts he committed within the community, but within his own family he enjoyed complete authority without appeal. Cato the Elder said: "He is the judge of his wife; his power has no limit; he can do what he wishes. If she has committed a fault, he punishes her; if she has drunk wine, he condemns her; if she has been guilty of adultery, he kills her." "Egnatius Metellus took a cudgel and beat his wife to death because she had drunk some wine. Not only did no one charge him with a crime, but no one even blamed him. Everyone considered this an excellent example of one who had justly paid the penalty for violating the laws of sobriety" (Valerius Maximus, 1st century A.D.). He had the same power over his children. Valerius Maximus reports matter-of-factly that Atilius killed his daughter because she was unchaste. As Edith Hamilton noted in *The Roman Way*, the Romans were proud of the popular story about Lucretia who committed suicide after she was raped because she was no longer chaste. In another popular story an "heroic" father killed his daughter rather than let her be a tyrant's mistress.

While studying ancient Rome, we see that the religious values of the city-state paralleled its legal values. As a result, since there was no common religion between people, families, or cities, there was no common law either, and no contract was binding. Furthermore, since neither the slave nor the stranger was part of the family unit, neither law nor religion applied to them. Laws based on religion were first instituted during the 8th century B.C. and were attributed to Romulus (753-716 B.C.). He compelled all citizens to rear every male child born, and the firstborn female. He also made it illegal to kill a child under three years of age, unless they were crippled or genetically deformed from birth. He allowed parents to expose such children provided they had first displayed them to their five nearest neighbors and had obtained their approval. Infanticide was part of the life of early Rome but was not as extensive as it later became.

Special laws were applied to foreigners. They could not be proprietors in Rome. They were not permitted to marry and if they did, the marriage was void and the children resulting from the union were considered bastards. A foreigner could not make a contract with a Roman citizen because the law would not recognize his part of the contract. Therefore he could not partake in commerce, he was not allowed to inherit from another citizen, nor was a citizen permitted to inherit from him. His only opportunity to participate in normal Roman life was to become a "client" of a citizen. Only by choosing a patron, and agreeing to be subject to that citizen's rule, could a foreigner take part in civilian life. Although he was not a free man, this option was far better than being labeled an enemy.

No mercy was granted to an enemy. A Roman considered it a glorious deed to assassinate an enemy soldier. In fact, around 170 B.C. General Paulus Aemilius sold as slaves 100,000 Epirots who had voluntarily surrendered to him. He promised them "just consideration." The "consideration" was to spare their lives.

These Romans of the Republic made war not only on enemy soldiers, but upon entire populations—men, women, children, and slaves. They burned fields and crops. Theirs was a classic scorched-earth policy, and their wars caused entire races of people to disappear while the land they had inhabited was turned to semidesert. Because of this policy—all done in the name of religion and family—the land and cities surrounding Rome were destroyed. The cities and nations farther away that accepted Roman dominance eventually were incorporated.

As years passed the Romans began to mix the plebeian and

foreign classes with their own population. The Romans were now related to all the peoples in the area—the Latins, Sabines, Etruscans, and Greeks, among them—and during the days of the empire, Romans were truly a mixture of several races with an assemblage of several worships. The rules against intermarriage no longer applied. It became the first cosmopolitan nation-state.

Rome was the only city-state that knew how to increase its population by war. Not only did the Romans have a scorched-earth policy, they now annexed all that they conquered and distributed it as farms and vineyards as rewards. They brought home the inhabitants of captured cities and gradually, over the generations, made Romans of them. They also sent colonists into conquered countries to spread Roman culture wherever possible. When Rome conquered a country and its people, it took that country's gods to Rome to possess their power for Rome but did not give the enemy Roman gods. Thus Rome, again through religion, became involved with the entire world.

Rome dealt with their conquered victims in a very organized way. Roman soldiers massacred the male population of their enemy lands and supplied a force of Roman soldiers to control the survivors. Then they sent a citizen into the country to manage it, giving him absolute authority over the province. In return, he sent tribute to Rome. However, the way he ran his province was entirely up to him: he could fix taxes, exert military control, and dispense justice; he was the living law. No provincial foreigner could appeal to Rome directly. He had to find a Roman citizen who would act as his patron, for he had no right to demand the protection of Roman law. It became common for these magistrates to embezzle public funds. Wars were fought, not only to protect the empire but to gain more money. Bribery and corruption took the apparent trappings of democracy and destroyed it.

The mass of people in the small city-states surrounding the city of Rome did not receive the benefits of Rome's armies' success, yet they were the ones supplying the armies with soldiers. Only the rich and aristocratic gained, winning more power, more land, and more wealth. As a result, there was an agrarian revolt, a civil war, that killed 300,000 people in central Italy over a three-year period. By 90 B.C. so few men were left to fight wars of self-protection or of conquest that all Italian freemen who swore allegiance to Rome were given citizenship instead of being killed.

For a long period there was one city that remained intact with its own institutions and laws, and that was Rome. Millions of people living in Roman city-states had no laws that were recognized or followed. Their laws were entirely those of the provincial governor. This state of chaos was controlled simply by force.

Gradually the conquered nations, after one or more generations, successively entered Rome, and more people gained Roman citizenship through their power and status. At one time the title "citizen of Rome" had been significant. It later became a common and unimportant term. Prior to the rise of Christianity, there was finally one single Roman country with one name, one government, and a single code of laws for all.

As we will see, the family structure—the strength of early Rome—lasted from about 500 to 200 B.C.,[19-21] though at no time during this period were women actually free. They could not marry without their father's consent, and even a married daughter remained under her father's authority unless he willingly gave it over to her husband (manumitted her). A woman could not appear in court, even as a witness. As a widow she could not claim rights to her husband's estate.

In the time of the later republic, women's rights were broadened.[22-25] Women were no longer confined to separate quarters; they ate with their husbands and his friends, though they were not permitted to recline, as the men did. This was psychologically significant since only freemen were allowed to recline.

Religious and festival activities included extensive sexual interplay. Still, all free Romans required the intact virginity of their young women, though not of men. A nonvirgin would have little opportunity for a reasonable marriage, or a life of prostitution was one prospect. Early in Roman history there were few female prostitutes, though there were many in the later days of the empire.

In the early period, men often married young for the purpose of having children. Children were considered economic assets on the small freeholding farms. At this time the minimum legal age for marriage was 14 for boys and 12 for girls.

But the small farm family unit gradually declined. Because these families had many children during this early period in Roman history, women were still an important part of the family unit. In 234 B.C. there were 270,713 citizens in Rome —all free adult males. By 189 B.C. there were 1,100,000, because the poor began moving into the city. South of the Rubicon—the stream that formed the border between Italy and Cisalpine Gaul—there was a population of approximately 5,000,000.

By Nero's time (54-68 A.D.),[26] the city had become almost unmanageable. The Empire was constantly at war and, because of increasing poverty in the countryside, there was a mass influx of people into the cities. The common people struggled to survive. Poverty, disease, and starvation wrought havoc. The central family unit began to disappear. It seemed that everything in Roman life had changed.

In fewer than 100 years, Rome had gone from a city of martial and democratic fervor to one of reckless luxury. The rich drank heavily and squandered their funds. Slavery was rampant. Male and female prostitution and homosexuality flourished. So prized were pretty male boys as sexual partners that men paid the price of a small farm to obtain one. Female prostitution became so extensive that Cato declared: "All other men rule over women; but we Romans, who rule all men, are ruled by our women."

By 195 A.D. women won the right to administer their dowries and control their own lives. They could divorce their husbands and not infrequently would poison them. Many women avoided having children. They began to fill their time with a variety of domestic activities. By 160 A.D. Polybius noticed such a decline in the population—also caused by infanticide[27-35]—that the state was unable to raise an army. Instead the government hired mercenaries and, as a result, foreign ethnic groups became the backbone of the Roman military.

Rome conquered Greece in 146 B.C., and adopted Greece's philosophical and social ideals, particularly those they found sexually gratifying. Thus we find more homosexuality in Roman life, and more reference to the educated, liberated prostitute, the *hetarai*.

With the increased wealth and loosening of morals, marriage vows became less important. Adultery became a normal occurrence. Most wealthy women married at least twice. Marriage and dowry became mechanical financial manipulations that had nothing to do with the relationship between two people. Many of the leaders of society were married five times. Children were seen as a nuisance that merely complicated the finances of marriage and property. Only the poor could "afford" to have children.

The poor often mutilated their children[36,37] to arouse pity while begging, as well as to elicit laughter in various public performances. Seneca observed that such mutilation of children was not wrong; "Look on the blind wandering about the streets leaning on their sticks, and those with crushed feet," he wrote, "and still again look on those with broken limbs. This one's without arms, that one has had his shoulder pulled down out of shape in order that his grotesqueries may excite laughter—let us go to the origin of all those ills—a laboratory for the manufacture of human wrecks—a tavern filled with the limbs torn from living children. What wrong has been done to the republic? On the contrary, have not these children been done a service inasmuch as their parents had cast them out?"

Soranus noted in 100 A.D. that the average time of weaning

for infants was from 12 to 24 months, while Macrobius in 400 A.D. recorded that the weaning was extended to about 35 months. This indicates that children were kept with wet nurses longer, and were rarely seen in the first few months of life by their real mothers.

Wet nursing became the rule, as few mothers wished to nurse their own children. In early Rome, parents acted as their children's educators. They taught the rules of the family, reverence for the gods, and the importance of instant obedience to authority. Mother was the primary teacher until age 7. At age 7 the boy was placed directly under the care of teachers, while girls remained at home with their mothers. A girl's education was cut short because she would be married by age 12 or 14. Her brother, meanwhile, would be his father's constant companion beginning at age 7, working at his side, particularly since the early Romans were farmers.

Later, when more households kept slaves, the father and son went in different directions, and indolence became the rule. The father's most important responsibility was to teach the boy to be a soldier. He taught his son not only to work on the farm, but how to use arms, proper military procedure, and the "manly" sports such as riding, wrestling, and boxing. Some schools were formed by educated slaves and beating was used as part of the training process. Juvenal, Martial, and Horace refer to the cruelty of their teachers in using the rod and the whip. Since no adequate literature was produced in Rome many wealthy families sent their sons to Athens to attend school. Thus Greece, although conquered, was the intellectual master of the world, and Greek became the language of Rome.

Child abuse in Rome was rampant. Horace described in his *Epodes* how a young boy was captured so his fresh liver could be used to make a love potion. Starvation of children was common, as noted by Plutarch. Even the emperors, in their autobiographies, admitted that in early childhood they were constantly hungry. Sexual abuse was also widespread, but occurred less frequently among the aristocratic boys only because they were protected by the pedagogues (slaves) who walked with them whenever they went outside. There were boy brothels in every city in the Empire, even after laws prohibited homosexuality with free boys. When free boys were not available, slave boys were kept for that purpose. Thus, it was not unusual for a free-born boy to see his father sleeping with, or having sexual relations with a slave boy his own age. Fathers did not hide this activity from their sons.

We also find that children were often sold into concubinage. Musonius Rufus (a philosophical writer) pondered whether there could be some justification for a boy to resist this abuse, but he drew no conclusions. He referred to one father who had a handsome male child and sold him to a brothel for a good profit. Plutarch referred to the gold ball freeborn boys sometimes wore around their necks so that men could tell they were free and were not available for sexual use.

Plutarch also referred to many instances of extensive sexual abuse of boys under 11 by their teachers and the pedagogues who were supposed to be protecting them. Laws were passed designed to limit the sexual attacks on schoolchildren by adults, but the legislation was never successful.

Quintilian, a teacher for many years in Rome, would often warn parents that their children were abused by other teachers. He used this as justification for not beating children while they were in school. Beatings could then be used as a threat to the child if he spoke about the sexual activity, or if he refused to participate sexually with his teachers. "When children are beaten, pain or fear frequently have results of which it is not pleasant to speak and which are likely to be a source of shame, a shame which unnerves and depresses the mind and leaves the child to shun and loathe the light. Further, if inadequate care is taken in the choices of respectable governors and instructors, I blush to mention the shameful abuse which scoundrels sometimes make of their right to administer corporal punishment or the opportunity not infrequently offered to others by the fear thus caused by the victims. I will not linger on this subject; there is more than enough if I have made my meaning clear."

Petronius, a historian who wrote around 50 A.D., noted how adults felt "the immature little tool of boys." He gave clear descriptions of the rape of a 7-year-old girl, with women clapping happily in a long line around the bed.

Quintilian referred to the widespread sexual debauchery[38-44] that took place in wealthy families, noting that sexual activity was observed by children and that they were invited to participate. Plutarch, in referring to sexual activity between older men and younger boys, was ambivalent, mentioning that Plato thought it advisable. An older man who would caress and love a young boy would aid his mental development through a loving relationship. In Rome, homosexual activity became as common as it was in Greece.

Suetonius[45] condemned Tiberius because he "taught children of the most tender years, who he called his little fishes, to play between his legs while he was in the bath. Those which were not yet weaned but were strong and hardy, he set to fellatio." Tacitus tells the same story.

Anal intercourse was more common than fellatio, and Martial gave written directions on how this activity should take place. In Imperial Rome there were *voluptates*—boys who had been castrated in the cradle so that they could be placed into brothels and sold to men for "buggering." Domitian, who reigned between 81 and 96 A.D., was the first emperor to pass a law prohibiting castration of infants for use in brothels.

Paulus Aegineta described a technique of castrating young boys, "since we are sometimes compelled against our will by persons of high rank to perform the operation—by compression is thus performed: children, still of a tender age, are placed in a vessel of hot water, and then when the parts are softened in the bath, the testicles are to be squeezed with the fingers until they disappear." Other techniques employed included surgical removal. Juvenal reports that doctors were often required to perform this operation. It was not uncommon for a small child to see castrated males. Many pedagogues, teachers, and prisoners were castrated.

Even though Constantine passed a law against castration, the practice continued because some parents believed it might advance their political ambitions by producing children to be used sexually by men or as court eunuchs. It was also done as a "cure" for a variety of diseases. And there were many "gelders" who wanted to obtain childrens' testicles for magical medical potions.

Castration was not the only abuse children faced. The literature of antiquity explains in detail how children's nightmares were treated by beating the child in order to drive the devil and demons out of its mind. In addition, frightening pictures of demons would be painted on walls. The parents' illogical reasoning was to keep children frightened so that they would not have nightmares to begin with.

L. deMause,[46] in *The History of Childhood*, points out that the children of ancient times were often physically or mentally retarded as a result of poor care. The restriction and filth of the swaddling—often children lay in their own excrement—and other cruel practices added to a child's general neglect. The index deMause used to study a child's health was the age at which the child began to walk. The normal age today is ten to twelve months, but children of ancient times usually walked later. He cites a report by Macrobius in 400 A.D. that children did not walk until 28 months. Today, a child who is not walking by 28 months is considered retarded or otherwise damaged; it is a significant sign of pathology. In fact, deMause considers the period of antiquity up to the 4th century A.D. as belonging to the "Infanticidal Mode" in his history of the evolution of childhood.

From 150 B.C. to 1 A.D. the power of the head of the Roman family diminished and the ancient family discipline and structure was completely destroyed. A Roman woman now moved about as freely as a man and, in some cases, for financial reasons, more freely. Women divorced their husbands as readily as men divorced their wives, and they participated freely in all the activities their money would allow.

Emperor Augustus[47] tried to deal with the extensive decrease in birthrate among the Romans (and the increase among the non-Romans) by encouraging Roman women to have more children rather than devoting their attention to making themselves sexually attractive. He made marriage obligatory for all males over 16 and women under 60. He exacted penalties for those who were celibate. Taxes were placed on those who had no children, with lower taxes on those who had more. Appointments to office were based on who had the largest family, and mothers with three or more children were given special powers and freedom from their husbands. However, all of these laws were unsuccessful. Men without children were courted by those who expected to inherit from them as their friends. As a general rule, Romans avoided marriage. Petronius' *Satyricon* demonstrates the distortions and corruption of Rome.

Originally children were reared because of the obligation, honor, and necessity of the family religion. Later, many people viewed the reproduction of children in a city that was crowded beyond endurance as absurd. Juvenal commented, "Nothing will so endear you to your friends as a barren wife." Instead of marrying, couples formed loose, temporary contracts for sexual and political needs. Women began taking eunuchs as contraceptive husbands. They entered into sham marriages with poor men who understood that no children were wanted but that extramarital lovers were acceptable. The population of children was controlled with contraception (both mechanical and chemical), extensive abortion, coitus interruptus, and infanticide. As Tacitus put it a hundred years later, "Marriages and the bearing of children did not become frequent, so powerful is the attraction of the childless state."

The decimation of the population of Rome due to infanticide, rampant abortion, and contraception tells us how the value of children declined from its early stages when the despotic father controlled the family. Though the Romans did not sacrifice children to the extent of the Carthaginians and various other cultures, they did sacrifice non-Romans when they felt threatened. In 225 B.C., when Rome was being pursued by a Carthaginian army, the Roman senate sacrificed two Gauls and two Greeks by burying them alive.

The Julian laws[48] designed to deter adultery, child prostitution, and to eliminate castration to produce eunuch slaves, were unsuccessful; these activities continued. With greater destruction of the home, wet nursing became the rule. Soranus, in the 1st century A.D., wrote: "One should, on the other hand, provide several wet nurses for the children who are to be nursed safely and successfully. For it is precarious for the nursling to become accustomed to one nurse who might become ill or die, and then, because of the change of milk, the child sometimes suffers from the strange milk and is distressed, while sometimes it rejects it altogether and succumbs to hunger."

We not only see abuse of women and children as routine and unremarked, but we also detect elements of gross disturbance in the society, such as cannibalism. "The story is that the daughters of Minyas (Leucippe, Arsinoe, and Alcathoe) went crazy. They developed a craving for human meat and drew lots to choose among their children. Leucippe won and offered up her son Hippasos to be torn to pieces" (Plutarch, 2nd century A.D.).

Killing a child was generally accepted; Pliny the Elder wrote of men who tried to improve their virility by eating the leg marrow and brain of an infant, and using part of its body for a love potion. This was common during the 1st century B.C., as recorded by Horace and others.

When the Emperor Diocletian[49] became ill in 303 A.D., the state required a general sacrifice. Anyone who did not sacrifice a child during the emperor's illness would be immediately executed.

Many stories were written of filial affection but the affection was always one-sided. The child took care of the parent. Boys and girls waited on their parents at the table, but were not permitted to eat with them.

Most children sacrificed to gods in Rome were killed by secret societies, such as that led by the priest Julianus, who killed many boys in secret magical rites. Suetonius wrote that for one year the senate decreed that no male children should be raised. They believed that an omen had warned them to issue this decree.

It was more common to kill the enemies' children than one's own—especially if the enemy child was of a royal stock. More royal infants were murdered than nonroyal. Philo reported: "Some of them do the deed with their own hands; or throw them into a river or into the depths of the sea, after attaching some heavy substance to make them sink more quickly under its weight. Others take them to be exposed on some deserted place hoping, they themselves say, that they may be saved, but leaving them in actual truth to suffer the most distressing fate. For all the beasts that feed on human flesh visit the spot and feast unhindered on the infants, a fine banquet provided by the sole guardians, those who above all other should keep them safe, their fathers and their mothers. Carnivorous birds, too, come flying down and gobble up the fragments."

The population of native Romans gradually dwindled, but there was no legislation to outlaw infanticide until 374 A.D. Even that did not stem the tide. Church leaders were more concerned about the parents' souls than the destruction of a child's life. St. Justin the Martyr reasoned that it was not right to expose children because a Christian might meet his own child later in a brothel and to have sexual relations with his offspring would be a sin. St. Justin's hypothesis did have some logical merit since many exposed children, male and female, were retrieved by strangers and turned into prostitutes.

In 449 A.D. it is reported that parents in Rome and Gaul sold their children through the use of middlemen to the Vandals. It is interesting to note that at the same period in history, the Germanic tribes had long established in their laws and in their culture various prohibitions against child murder. Similar humane laws did not come to the Roman Christian world until 100 years later.

It was not until 787 A.D. that the first asylum was founded for the care of abandoned infants. The statistics for children during this early period indicate that infanticide and abandonment continued well into the Middle Ages.

In desperation Emperor Augustus[50] tried another approach. He banned Egyptian (Ptolemaic) and Asiatic cults from Rome since these nations practiced infanticide as part of their cultures, with the exception of the Jews, since they were so family oriented and were considered a positive influence.

The only residents of Rome who did not intermarry were the Jews.[51] By 59 B.C. there were 20,000 Jews in the capital, who remained separate from their neighbors, scorning polytheism and idol worship. Their morals were seen as severe. They refused to attend theaters or games, particularly those that involved murder, moral licentiousness, and other acts they deemed inhumane. Some were rich, but many were not, and they continued to be a unit in the Roman community that remained different from all the others. Juvenal denounced their fertility and Tacitus their monotheism. However, many educated Romans admired the Jews' monotheism and sought to be converted. A number of the most influential Roman families observed the Jewish Sabbath as a day of worship and rest. As Will Durant[10] noted, ". . . with its influx of people from the Orient, etc. into Rome, the fertile conquered became masters in the sterile master's house."

During the Empire (45 B.C. to 460 A.D.) an increased decline in morals becomes readily apparent from the barbaric forms of entertainment. The emperors Nero and Caligula encouraged many grossly sadistic activities as diversion for the masses. Condemned criminals were dressed in animal skins and thrown into arenas with ravenous wild beasts. Sometimes plays were written in which a condemned man was forced to play a famous tragic role, and was killed before the audience. Some "actors" were burned to death, publicly castrated, or forced to hold their hands over burning coals. Women were forced to have sexual relations with animals or to fight armed men. Any combatant who was reluctant to die was prodded with hot irons.

A police state developed spies, informers, and the ruthless execution of anyone who interfered, or whose property the state wished to confiscate. The depreciation of women and children was seen as "entertainment." Young girls were raped and forced to have intercourse with animals, small children suspended by their legs from poles so that hyenas could pull them down and eat them alive.

Many committed suicide to avoid this public torture. In the spectacles given by Augustus, 10,000 men might take part in a mock battle. Following a battle, attendants went into the arena dressed like Charon and probed the fallen gladiators with sharp rods. If they were feigning death they were hit on the head with a mallet.

It is significant that these atrocities were completely acceptable; these "games" were so much a part of everyday life that Juvenal, who denounced everything else, did not denounce them. Pliny the Younger, considered highly civilized for his day, praised the Emperor Trajan for providing such spectacles to "compel men to be noble and scorn death."

Rome in its imperial period moved toward an excess of sensuality. The Roman idea of love was purely sexual. Lust was the rule for everything: sex, food, or violence. Orgies and feasts lasted for days. There was a limit to how much sex one could participate in, but there was no end to the eating orgies. Battles were fought with food—expensive and exotic food. The idea was to see how much one could consume. Those who overindulged were carried to a vomitarium to regurgitate and return to the contest of the table, gorging on rare delicacies, reclining on a couch.[52] Of course, this was not the life of the poor Roman citizen, who lived on grain paste, coarse bread, and a porridge made from millet and polluted water. Occasionally they were able to obtain a small piece of fish, olives, beans, or figs.

There was such a severe shortage of food in Rome[53] in 70 A.D. that if the ships that brought food to the city were late in arriving, there would be panic in the city among the poor and hungry. Even when there was food, cooking was a problem because there was a fuel shortage in the city as well, and most food was eaten raw.

Another victim of Roman society was the slave. At first, during the monarchical period there were very few slaves and most were treated with relative consideration because they were valuable to their owner. However, slaves were essentially treated like property. In the early republic, a creditor could imprison a defaulting debtor in his own private dungeon and sell him into slavery—even kill him for not paying his debt.

As the Romans conquered and enslaved much of the world, poverty increased in the lands around Rome. This caused an enormous influx of slaves to pour into Rome and its various cities. Rome was no longer an agricultural community. To survive, the increasing population of the city relied on the importation of food, on plunder, and internal slavery. Wars were fought to gain slaves. The commerce of the city was built on the business of slavery. It was not unusual for as many as 10,000 slaves to be auctioned off in a single day in one of the many slave markets. By 104 B.C., only 2000 Roman citizens actually owned property. According to Appian, the condition of the poor "became even worse than before. The plebeians lost everything. The lot of citizens and soldiers continued to decline."

During the period from 14 A.D. to 96 A.D., Seneca observed that the wealthy controlled the land, where they cultivated olive orchards and vineyards. The poorest soil was left for food crops. Just as in Greece, where the lands were turned over for commercial purposes and the people could not manage except by working for someone else, slavery had become the mode of survival.

Beloch (the historian) estimated that around 30 B.C. there were 400,000 slaves in Rome proper—approximately half the population. The population of Italy was 1.5 million. By comparison, in Pergamum, in ancient Mysia in western Asia Minor, a fourth of the population were slaves in 170 A.D.

Of those employed in industry and trade 80% were slaves, and most of the mail and clerical work in the government was performed by public slaves. Slaves were everywhere in the environment, and were an intrinsic part of people's lives. Young slave boys and small children were used as sexual amusement. There were markets in Rome where one could buy deformed slaves as entertainment. It was customary for household slaves (many of them women) to be beaten and occasionally killed, since their individual value was so low. Nero's father killed his freed men, even though they were no longer slaves, because they refused to drink as much as he wanted them to. A freed man (by purchase or as a gift) was still subject to many of the rules of slavery, even into the third generation.

Nero[54] himself was no better than his father, and was among the more degenerate of the emperors. He often disguised himself and visited brothels, roamed the streets with his comrades, robbed shops, insulted women, raped boys, and murdered. A senator who was approached in one of these marauding adventures and who defended himself too vigorously against the disguised emperor was forced afterwards to kill himself by the emperor's order. When Nero was 22 he killed his mother in justifiable fear that she might poison him. Even the brilliant Seneca, who tried to teach Nero and control him, was eventually forced by Nero to commit suicide. Before he died Seneca described the sadistic Roman practice of torture and abuse of slaves.

The slave had no legal rights and was neither called nor considered a man. The rights of the master were absolute. A slave was the master's property to hurt, destroy, or injure in any way he wished. If a slave retaliated and killed a master, then, according to law, all other slaves owned by that master had to be put to death. Emperor Hadrian (117-138 A.D.) was among the few who tried to modify conditions by making it a criminal offense to mutilate a slave for sexual purposes, but he was unsuccessful. Marcus Aurelius (161-180 A.D.) encouraged slave owners to bring errant slaves before the courts rather than to punish them themselves, but this also failed. It was Roman dependence on slavery that helped contribute to the downfall of their empire.

During the last hundred years of the republic and throughout the empire, freeborn citizens who were not soldiers were either slaveholders or idle. The early Roman virtues of simplicity, legality, and temperance declined markedly and rapidly with the increase of slavery. Even the poorest gentleman citizen had ten slaves, some citizens as many as 20,000. Entire cities and nations of men, women, and children would be sold into slavery when conquered. When not useful for either labor or as sexual objects, they were killed.

When the number of slaves became too high and caused a financial burden, they were killed. This was sometimes accomplished by bringing them to Rome to be destroyed for the amusement of the Roman population. The heads of thousands of slaves were used as decoration around the Roman forum. Murder was an appreciated part of the everyday Roman life among even the most sophisticated Roman citizens.

In the late empire[55] a law was passed that changed the status of slaves from objects to people. As a result, fewer were sold for the purpose of fighting wild beasts in the amphitheater, and slaves could no longer could be put to death because they were too old or ill to work. But Romans found many loopholes in this new law. Roman law had a long and complicated history that was increasingly protective of its citizens in its writing, but never approached the benign attitudes of the Athenians toward their slaves, or the justice of the Hebrews. Even with the improved status of the legal system in Rome as the empire advanced, the law was essentially useless because of widespread corruption. It was almost impossible effectively to control the population. Romans used the principle of terror, the "long arm of Rome," to keep the citizenry in line. They killed to control. Suetonius, the Roman historian who lived from about 69 A.D. to about 140 A.D., noted that when the Romans took Perugia during one of many Italian civil wars, 300 prisoners of the patrician rank were offered as human sacrifices on the Ides of March at the altar of the god Junius.

Roman emperors,[56] to protect themselves and their offices, slaughtered potential enemies, commoners and men of authority alike, without trial or legal process. Thus, the various families that had been important in the history of Rome were eventually decimated.

Slaves were commonly beaten with sticks and lashed for minor offenses. In fact, flogging was a legal preliminary to every Roman execution and only women, Roman senators, and soldiers were exempt from it. A short whip (*flagrum*) was used, with braided leather thongs that had small iron balls and sharp pieces of sheep bone attached at intervals. The victim would be stripped of his clothing and, to make the beating easier for the master, the victim's hands were tied to an upright post. He was flogged across his back and buttocks until he reached a weakened state just short of collapse or death. The metal balls and sheep bones would bruise the muscle and tear the subcutaneous tissue and skin, causing damage to the muscle tissue and extensive bleeding.

The most extreme punishment of all was crucifixion,[57] a painful, lingering, and horrible death. Crucifixion was a punishment designed originally by the Persians, and later introduced to Egypt and Carthage by Alexander the Great. The Romans perfected the punishment, making it an even slower and more agonizing death than the one their predecessors had devised.

The condemned man carried the top half of a cross (*patibulum*) which weighed 75 to 125 pounds. To prolong the pain the Romans attached a horizontal wooden block or plank—like a small seat—affixed midway down the vertical (*stipes*). The victim's wrists were nailed to the crossbar and a nail was driven through his ankles.

The length of survival ranged from three hours to four days, depending on how much damage the whip had done. Insects would burrow into the open wounds and the eyes and ears of the dying victim. Birds of prey would tear at the wounds as well.

Most of the pain of crucifixion was the difficulty the victim had in breathing. Each respiration would be agonizing, and death would finally result from the loss of blood or asphyxiation. Death by crucifixion was excruciating (*excruciatus*, or "out of the cross"). Those crucified along the Appian Way would beg travelers to take pity and drive a lance through their heart.

By the late empire, all work that had been done by free persons of the lowest class, such as civil service, was now performed exclusively by slaves. It was the law.

In fact, Rome had an extensive body of laws designed to maintain the empire; however, they were rarely obeyed. Nonetheless, looking at the law will help us to identify the social problems that prevailed and to understand the philosophy of the legislators.

The law of the Twelve Tables, written around 450 B.C., about 50 years after the republic was established, changed Rome from a theocracy, where a deity was recognized as supreme ruler, to a form of democracy. Increasingly, lawyers replaced priests in Roman life. The law of the Twelve Tables—primitive rules whose object was to establish a societal norm—remained the basic law of Rome for approximately 900 years, and was the base upon which all other laws in the Roman Empire were written. The Twelve Tables were severe in character and retained some of the cruel power of the omnipotent father to "scourge, chain, imprison, sell, or kill any of his children." They decreed, among other statutes, that a son sold three times was thereafter free of his father's rule; patricians could not marry plebeians; and creditors had every right against a debtor, including his person. Death was decreed for even minor crimes and brutal tortures were the general rule.

In 117 A.D., Hadrian[58] attempted to organize the body of laws based on the Twelve Tables into the Perpetual Edict, to be observed by all judges of the Roman Empire. In his edict Hadrian took the right of the father to kill his son from the father and transferred it to the courts. He also established an extensive civil service. Hadrian was one of Rome's best and most effective emperors, though he did participate extensively in homosexual activities with children. Other emperors who followed him tried to liberalize the law, equalize the penalties for adultery for men and woman, and deprive ruthless masters of their slaves.

Marcus Aurelius,[59] the Philosopher Emperor, ruled well but left a son, Commodus, who destroyed everything he had created. Commodus drank, gambled, wasted public funds, and kept a harem of 300 women and 300 boys, often dressing in women's clothes at public games. Even the Romans considered him cruel. Emperor Antonius (138-161 A.D.) decreed that cases of doubt should be resolved in favor of the accused and that a man would be held innocent until proven guilty—a vital new addition. He also prohibited fathers' selling their sons into slavery and, by the 2nd century A.D., women were completely freed, after the age of 25, from subservience to their fathers. By 160 A.D. marriages required the consent of the woman as she could not be completely controlled by her father. A wife was given more rights in her dowry. However, by this time there was so much corruption that Antonius' law was ineffective. Not until the 4th century A.D. would any law or public opinion condemn infanticide.

There were many examples of more advanced laws in surrounding lands to which the Romans could have turned, but they derided them. The Roman magistrates and the educated population laughed at the Jewish law in Deuteronomy that gave privileges and protection to slaves and servants whether they were Israelites or heathen. They jeered at the concept of a Sabbath day of rest, and considered it superstitious. The Romans also rejected the sixth commandment, "Thou shall not kill." These humane laws were at odds with Roman life. Roman leaders could not comprehend that a child's life was as sacred as an adult's. Tacitus laughed at this concept.

Conclusion

Unfortunately, the observation of Gibbon[60] in his epic study, *The Decline and Fall of the Roman Empire*, can most specifically be applied to the Roman's treatment of children. He said: "The experience of past faults, which may sometimes correct the mature age of an individual, is seldom profitable to the success of generations of mankind."

Throughout Rome's history we see a gradual development of the Roman's relationship to families and women. At the outset, women were oppressed and fathers had the right to destroy their children or to sell them. Conditions progressed to a point when children and wives were given more freedom and greater consideration by law. In the later periods of the Roman Empire there was a breakdown of the family unit because of increasing adultery, harlotry, and general immorality.

Early Rome was an aristocracy, not a republic. It was a militaristic society with some checks and balances and a division of power that occasionally dissolved into mob rule. The Empire reached its height of power as luxury and sexual license replaced the organization of the family unit.

Though the Roman was a pragmatist in many ways, he also

acted somewhat paradoxically: he was wanton in the killing of his neighbors not of his religion; strict in his own practice of his religion as he lived out his entire day.

The Roman Empire, which lasted about 500 years, was in constant turmoil. Internally, it was depraved in its degradation of women, abuse of children, and torture of slaves. Its culture was based on feeding and satisfying the desires of the wealthy to the exclusion of all others. Externally, Rome was constantly fearful of civil war, outside enemies, slave revolts, and even of their own cruel dictators. Rome's eventual decay and collapse seems to have been its inevitable fate.

Chapter 6

China: East Meets West

> *An emperor knows how to govern when poets are free to make verses, people to act plays, historians to tell the truth, ministers to give advice, the poor to grumble at taxes, students to learn lessons aloud, workmen to praise their skill and seek work, people to speak of anything, and old men to find fault with everything.*
>
> Address of the Duke of Shao to King Li-wang, 845 B.C.

The dirt-walled villages that speckle the countryside are the life-blood of the ancient Chinese civilization. In these villages family life and morality is strong and specific. Life is precious, though at times it is not easy.

As we enter the village through a stone gate we see men and their sons scratching at the dry earth (*loess*) which has been scorched by drought. The year is 800 B.C.

Each family—and there are many here attending their small and meager plots—depends on the bounty of nature for life. Life goes on almost exclusively within the village walls, where boys will grow to be men in the image of their fathers. Girls will learn the fundamental duties of their lot. Laws, religion, respect, and family life are vital and governed by simple men with grand ideals.

This is China,[A] many small family (clan) communities in a vast unchanging cohesive fabric, that seemingly will last forever.

129

China is divided laterally by two main rivers, the Yellow and the Yangtze. The countryside is mostly mountainous with plains, some vast deserts, as well as a relatively small percentage of truly fertile areas. From the north and northeast flows the Liao River from Manchuria to the northeastern shore of the country. At the southwestern shore is the mouth of the Yellow River, which originates in the distant mountains of Shantung. To the north is the vast North China plain and far to the west is the great desert. From the Tibetan mountains flows the Yellow River, while the Yangtze originates in Szechuan province and flows north and west of Shanghai into the Pacific. China is cut up by mountain ranges into relatively isolated regions.

The climatic changes are even more extensive than the geographic ones. In the far west is Tibet, a high frozen desert with nomadic peoples, the Mongolian steppe, and the Tarim basin, which is an arid grassland. These are the grassy steppes of the Manchurian plain. The warmer, less arid regions in north central China have fertile soil but little rainfall. Periodic flooding irrigates the land. North of this is extremely rich land where little fertilization is needed because of the rich organic quality of the soil. This area is the origin of Chinese agriculture and civilization.

In the lower Yangtze Valley to the east and farther south is the rice growing area. Here the climate is warm and wet—completely distinct from the dry cold area of the northwest. The Szechuan basin in the west is a densely populated and very fruitful area. Of course, it includes the hot plateau of the southernmost area, which is subtropical and has a very high humidity level.

The annual flooding of China's fertile area by its rivers, especially the Yellow, was a mixed blessing in ancient times. Not only did it fertilize and irrigate, it also inundated and destroyed everything in its path. Its riverbed wandered hundreds of miles from any given location. Each year it deposited more of the richly organic soil wherever it passed, sometimes raising the level of the riverbed above the surface of the land. Any diking in ancient times could be disastrous due to sudden bursting and flooding of the lower lands. It is not surprising that the Yellow River bears the eponym "China's Sorrow."

This land that the Chinese call the "Middle Flowery Kingdom" is hemmed in by the highest mountains in the world, the largest ocean and one of the most extensive desert systems (the Gobi). These were natural divisions that the Chinese used well.

Western historians agree that China recorded its own history more accurately than any civilization the world has ever known. Its official historians have reported in careful detail since at least 776 B.C.

As a result of these records we have learned that the earliest dynasties were the Yao and Shun. The most enduring was the Chou, which was composed of 1700 principalities. Laws were codified by the Cheng in 535 B.C. (Chou-Li or Law of Chou). Emperors held their power by virtue of their piety, birth, and training, as well as their ability to administer the office of state. The common people farmed, lived in patriarchal families, and enjoyed considerable civil rights. Public affairs were determined by administrators of the state (six ministries) who controlled the activities and lives of the people and of the emperor.

By the 11th century B.C. (Yin dynasty) there was an advanced culture with an established aristocracy whose people tried to control the wandering Yellow River by diking it, building canals, and draining marshes. They developed the art of writing, and had a state religion with capitals, temples, and state halls. The Chinese peasants were cattle breeders and developed an extensive agricultural system. Evidence shows that there was a large organized population with an army divided into units of 3000 (9th century B.C., Chou) and that they had a judicial system with traveling magistrates.

The table of chronology on the next page encapsulates the history of the Chinese civilization.

There is little archaeological material available from the ear-

Chronology of Chinese Civilization

Legendary rulers	2852 B.C.	Ideographic writing begun.
Yao dynasty	2356-2255 B.C.	
Shun dynasty	2255-2205 B.C.	
Shang dynasty (Yin)	1766-1123 B.C.	Society changed from matriarchy to patriarchy.
Early Tang dynasty	1766-1753 B.C.	
Chou dynasty (Yin)	1122-255 B.C.	Thousand-volume encyclopedia produced.
Feudal Period	770-255 B.C.	
Lao-tze	604-517 B.C.	
Confucius	551-478 B.C.	
Period of the Warring States	403-221 B.C.	First compass invented.
Chin dynasty unification	255-206 B.C.	
Han dynasty	206 B.C.-221 A.D.	Ink is invented.
Tartar invasion	200-400 A.D.	
Later Tang dynasty	618-905 A.D.	Movable type invented.
Northern Sung dynasty	968-1127 A.D.	Gunpowder used in defense.
Tartars sack Kaifeng	1126 A.D.	
Southern Sung dynasty	1127-1279 A.D.	
Genghis Khan	1162-1227 A.D.	
(Yuan-Mongol dynasty)	1260-1368 A.D.	
Ming dynasty restoration	1368-1644 A.D.	
Ching (Manchu) dynasty	1644-1912 A.D.	

liest period in Chinese history because in 221 B.C. the man who called himself "First Emperor of China" (Chin) tried to destroy all remnants of past history so that all history would begin with him. He also slaughtered all scholars and historians who might have recorded material. The only scholars and books he did not destroy were those about medicine, agriculture, and forestry.

From archaeology, we know that humans have been living

in the area of central China for 400,000 years, with 4000 years of fairly well-recorded history and a well-established neolithic population center by 12,000 B.C. By 2500 B.C. China had a large population with thousands of villages, an agricultural economy, textiles, carpentry, and ceramics.

During the 18th century B.C. the populace practiced family and ancestor worship, as well as human sacrifice. Slaves were buried alive at royal burials, a practice which lasted until the Chin dynasty. By 500 B.C. there was such extensive intellectual development that there were more than 100 schools of philosophy.

Periods of social upheaval were marked by great intellectual development, with advancement in crafts, irrigation, agriculture, and marketing. Theirs was an intense money-based economy. For example, the crossbow, an early Chinese invention, was later perfected—built of iron and developed into one of the ancients' primary weapons.

The first Chinese dictionary, written in 1500 B.C., had 40,000 characters. Long before Pythagoras, the triangular theories were known in China. And by 1000 B.C. the complete structure of Chinese script had been developed—the same that is used today—and a textbook compiled in mathematics which included square roots, geometry, algebra, and a theory of motion.

The only man-made creation that can be seen from space by today's astronauts is the 1500-mile-long Great Wall of China, built between 356 and 215 B.C. Even the greatest architectural achievement of the West, the pyramids of Egypt, shrink by comparison. The Great Wall was intended to slow the approach of invaders and to give the Chinese army time to assemble and repel the attack. This technique succeeded for centuries. The wall was wide enough to carry two chariots across, and had many towers and turrets.

Despite myths to the contrary, Europe was discovered by China. During the Han dynasty, Chang Ch'hien was sent to Bactria and established the famous silk trade routes that went from China into Iran.

Parthia (Iran) monopolized its valuable relationship with China, acting as the sole source of communication between the Romans and Chinese. Parthians told Chinese emissaries stories of the terrible, "barbaric" activity in Rome, convincing them that contact with the Romans would contaminate the Chinese civilization. At the time the Chinese were making extensive progress in astronomy, calculation of the calendar, geology, botany, and chemistry. The Chinese had an extensive bibliographic reference system for experts in every field. They had even developed the use of paper. Their technology in ceramics and textiles was so well refined that it has not been equaled in the West until recently. They became masters of the sea with the invention of a rudder, and no people could equal their naval exploits in the 1st century A.D.

Despite a series of wars with groups who were threatened by its cultural advances and expansion, the Chinese always kept their ambition and their drive to succeed technologically. For example, during the Sui dynasty (550-671 A.D.) the Chinese tried to build an extensive inland water transportation system, the Grand Canal. They employed 5.5 million people, aged 15 to 55, and supervised them with 50,000 police. Every fifth family had to contribute one person to the project, in addition to supplying and preparing food for them. Theoretically, 2 million men died in the project. Much of this project remains, where it has not been destroyed by floods and other causes.

In battles with the Moslems, Chinese paper makers were captured in the Battle of Samarkand and forced to teach paper manufacturing to the Arabs. Later this invention was passed on to Europe. Throughout its history ancient China was the largest and the most disciplined of all its neighbors in the sciences and arts. They were masters of shipbuilding, architecture, weaponry, medicine, pharmacology, chemistry, ceramics, astronomy, mathematics, metallurgy, archaeology, and biology. Developments in these fields passed quickly from east to west (originally trading—and, later the transmission of the knowledge of plants) with such products as oranges, pears, peaches, roses, peonies, azaleas, camellias, chrysanthemums, silk, lacquer boxes, pottery, ceramics, ivory carvings, spices, and an early form of steel known as seric iron. It seems certain that the Arabs' advance in mathematics and astronomy was due to their extensive contact and communication with the Chinese.

Despite its scientific advancement[1-4] and tight organization, hardly a decade passed in ancient China without warfare against barbarians who were constantly pressing in from the frontier. This warfare and conflict between the various states in the early period of China's history led to as many as 36 kings during a 200-year span, a time of anarchy known as the "Warring States."

Through it all the peasants continued to keep their distance from much of the fighting and political maneuvering of the warring factions. The soldiers were volunteers who could not function on the farms, or conscripts. When the warfare ceased, the Chinese were able to expand domestic trade. This trade resulted in the growth of a strong middle class that wore leather shoes, silk clothing, rode in carts, and traveled the country by an extensive network of canals. Middle-class homes were more sophisticated than the homes of their contemporaries in Solon's Greece, with tables, chairs, plates, dishes, ornamental pottery, and other refined amenities.

In addition to widespread material growth, the Chinese produced some great thinkers, among them Lao-Tze (604-517 B.C.), whose book the *Tao-Te-Ching* (the Book of the Way, and the Book of Virtues) was probably the most important in Chinese history. "The Way" (Tao) is the way of nature, the way of living wisely, the proper road of life. "The Way" is to be found by rejecting extraneous elements in life and living modestly.

Confucius (K'ung-fu-tze) was another important philosopher. In his view, "A man's character was formed by the Odes, developed by the Rites, and perfected by music." He used the

Socratic method long before Socrates. The five volumes Confucius left were added to four previous books written by other philosophers. Together they constituted the Nine Classics in Chinese literature.

According to Confucius: "When the Great Principle (or the Great Similarity) prevails, the whole world becomes a republic; they elect men of talents, virtue and ability; they talk about sincere agreement and cultivate universal peace. Thus men do not regard as their parents only their own parents, nor treat as their own children only their own children . . . each man has his rights, and each woman her individuality safeguarded." The practicality of Confucian philosophy satisfied the Chinese and became the foundation for administering the country. The naturalistic philosophy of Taoism, meanwhile, became the way of functioning within the family.

Shih Huang-ti, the illegitimate son of a queen of Chin, began the unification of China in 221 B.C. As a result of his military efforts, the Huns were unable to conquer China and moved into Europe and Italy. We may say that Rome fell because China built a wall.

The Han dynasty, which followed the Chin, lasted 400 years and gave its name to the Chinese ethnic group. All Chinese consider themselves Han, with the exception of 3% to 7% of the population whom they consider foreign. This is an expression of their xenophobia. The Han restored freedom of speech and writing and pursued a policy of peace. However, they did manage to push back the barbarians who were a constant threat, and to extend their rule over all of China, Korea, Manchuria, Annam, Indochina, and Turkestan. This rule was not oppressive and passed on their higher culture. Under the Han dynasty civil service expanded and the Imperial library grew to house 3100 volumes on the classics, 2700 on philosophy, 1300 on poetry, 2500 on mathematics, 870 on medicine, and 790 on general information.

One Han emperor tried to abolish slavery and divide some

of the land of the wealthy among the peasants, but he was unsuccessful. Between 200 and 400 A.D., the Tartars invaded and conquered China but were absorbed into Chinese civilization. The Tartars were followed by the Tang. Emperor Tai Tsung (627-650 A.D.) told the people: "If I diminished expenses, lighten the taxes, and do away with dishonest officials so that the people have clothing enough, this will do more to abolish robbery than the employment of the severest punishment." By this time the Imperial library had grown to 54,000 volumes and China was undoubtedly the most powerful, enlightened, progressive, and best governed empire on earth.

Emperor Ming Huang (the "Brilliant Emperor") reigned from 713 to 756 A.D. He abolished capital punishment and reformed the court system, but levied heavy taxes on the people. Though he encouraged poets, scholars, and artists, and established the college of music, he ended his reign in dissolute luxury and subject to the whims of a young concubine, Yang Kwei-fei.

The Tang dynasty was followed by a period of upheaval with five dynasties in 53 years. Finally the Sung dynasty was established on a platform that "the state should take the entire management of commerce, industry, and agriculture into its own hands, with a view to succoring the working classes and prevent it from being ground into dust by the rich." Again there was a rapid advance in sciences, literature, philosophy, and the arts.

By 1000 A.D., with the aid of book printing, the entire saga of Chinese history was compiled in a 5000-volume set. Hundreds of these sets were printed and copies still exist today.

From the Sung dynasty through the Ming dynasty scholarship dominated the Chinese civilization. As American historian Will Durant[5] wrote: "The pursuit of wisdom and the passion of beauty are the two poles of the Chinese mind, and China might loosely be defined as philosophy and porcelain." Further, it was his view that: "Until it began to yield its own ideas to Western influence, China refused to recognize any distinction between the artist and the artisan, or between the artist and the workers; nearly all industry was manufacture and all manufacture was handicraft; industry, like art, was the expression of personality and things . . . China excelled every country in artistic taste and the multiplication of beautiful objects for daily use."

Sculpture was a minor art as was architecture for homes, though for major projects such as the Great Wall and the extensive construction of canals, it was obviously a well developed science. Because many of the buildings were made of wood, there are few remains from ancient times. Durant believes that Chinese architecture did not develop because the civilization lacked a hereditary aristocracy, "a powerful priesthood, and a strong, wealthy central government." A very top-heavy (moneyed) oligarchy lends itself to self-aggrandizing monuments, not characteristic of China.

Chinese peasant homes were modest, made of wood, or pounded dirt, with rarely any stone above the foundation level. The homes were single-story and rested on posts with a wooden frame about the entire base, with few windows and little glass. Projecting eaves kept the rain out and heat was from portable braziers. Being cold in the winter was common to all, and the Chinese wore much padded clothing.

Genghis Khan conquered China (12th century), but attempted to rule it without Sinicizing the Mongols, placing the Mongols in the highest positions of office. But they could not run the massive country without the involvement of Chinese civil servants. By the time of Kublai Khan (the grandson of Genghis Khan) the Chinese managed to absorb the Mongols, and shortly thereafter the Mongols fell to the Ming and their great restoration (1368 A.D.). After 277 years the Ming dynasty was overthrown by the Manchus (1644 A.D.), who ultimately gave China one of the most prosperous and peaceful periods in its history. But the Manchu dynasty also introduced a distinct cultural phobia regarding discussion of sexual material and an even greater xenophobia than had ever before existed.

China, compared to its contemporary civilizations, was not only huge in area, but in population with, in 280 B.C., about 14 million people, twice the number in the entire Mediterranean world. In 200 A.D. there were 28 million Chinese, by 726 A.D. 41.5 million, and by 1644, 90 million. By the 14th century A.D. there were 200 cities in China, each larger and more sophisticated than Venice, then considered the most important city in the western world.

Their written language, which could be read by all Chinese, no matter what their dialect, helped solidify the vast Chinese civilization. Since the written language has endured, anyone knowing the Chinese language today can basically decipher historical documents that are more than 2000 years old.

In reading Chinese history we are impressed by the resiliency of the people and the cohesiveness of their culture. But the Chinese took these cultural patterns for granted. They never believed that their emperors were permanent or that their dynasties would last forever. Rather, they would say the dynasties only existed as long as "heaven above and the people below wanted it to last." Yet they had an unshakable belief in the permanence of their race and their culture.

Chinese society was based on a mixture of a naturalistic religion, morals, and philosophy. Traditionally the culture had three guides for behavior: Tao, Filial Piety, and Face, which shaped the actions and personality of the civilization from ancient times to the present. Tao, or the Heavenly Way, embodied the laws and patterns of nature and society from which every man was expected to mold his thoughts and behavior. The Yin and Yang were related respectively to male and female in the cosmic force and were contained in each person. In the circular movement of life, when Yang was at its maximum it changed into Yin. When Yin reached its maximum it changed into Yang, for Yang harbors a Yin element and Yin harbors a Yang element. Every man had a feminine element and every woman a masculine one. For this reason, man and woman required each other.

Taoist philosophy required free sexual communication between man and woman. In this philosophy the woman was venerated because she was closer to the forces of nature, since new life came from her womb. It was also believed that the woman's body contained elements indispensable for a man to be a man. One could not follow the supreme order and follow the way of Tao without sexual union with a woman.

The Chinese worshiped their ancestors. They held a Confucian concept of a vague heaven filled with great ancestors. All organized religions were tolerated in China. There were no religious wars. A Chinese could find himself animistic, Taoist, Buddhist, and a Confucianist all at the same time. He considered nothing certain. And, as if he were humoring someone else's beliefs, he would sometimes pay a priest a modest sum to say prayers over his grave. Despite 1000 years of Christian proselytizing and 1200 years of extensive contact with the Moslem world, fewer than 1% of the population was converted to either religion.

Instead, the Chinese loved to compromise. That way they saved their own faces and the faces of the enemy. At all social levels they were not violent in speech or in manners. They were clean, sober, generally peaceable and kindly, neighborly, thrifty, industrious, unassuming people. Yet they were surprisingly rigid in their hatred of criminals and warriors. They were honest in their commerce, except with barbarians, whom they felt neither deserved nor required such honesty in trading. They were not individualists, but collectivistic, bureaucratic, and prone to group activity. They wished only to interweave their lives with ancient custom.

A significant aspect of Chinese family life[(B)] was their worship of ancestors, whom the ancient Chinese believed could affect a person's life in the spirit world. This belief encouraged good behavior, which prolonged life, while bad behavior shortened it. At death, a person's spirit was believed to pass through a series of judgments at which the ancestors assisted. A person who behaved badly in life would be submitted to torture in death. At the court of the tenth judge the spirit was judged for potential reincarnation. Those who failed this judgment were destined to eternal damnation, would possibly be reincarnated as lower animals or, at best, peasants.

The judges (deceased former clan heads) evaluated individual spirits of the recently deceased for their industry, frugality, honesty, and harmony. The greatest virtue was filial piety. A good person would have been kind to the aged, helped the community, honored teachers, and shown piety to the gods. The wealthy person was expected to have helped build public bridges and roads, established schools, and explained scriptures and sacred books to the ignorant.

In the most ancient periods the Chinese had extensive mourning rituals. For a three-year mourning period coarse cloth was worn with the edges torn. According to the *Book of Harmony* by Zhougong,[6,7] the two things necessary to achieve the harmony, filial piety and fraternal affection, must be demonstrated by proper mourning. The closer the kinship to the father/son relationship, the greater the expression of sorrow. However, more sorrow was shown for the mother by the son (3 years) than when the father died (2 years). This is a clear indication that the Chinese knew that the feelings of mother and child were the most powerful and needed acknowledgment in mourning, despite the official statement of the first importance of the father/son relationship. The social show of mourning included public crying and wailing, with a disregard for personal comfort and appearance in wearing the coarsest clothes until the mourning period was over.

Dead parents, of course, became ancestors who kept watch over the family. There were two types of ancestor worship, domestic and extradomestic. The only universal worship was for the so-called kitchen god, a supernatural inspector of the household sent by the emperor of heaven. His responsibility was to watch over household life and report to a superior each year. His report would determine the fortunes of the household.

The extradomestic worship applied to the clan as a whole.[8] Tablets were placed in a clan temple for each clan ancestor and prayers were offered to them. Despite appearances, the concept and worship of the powerful ancestor was not a driving force among the ancient Chinese. Much more significant was their devotion to their house god.

Since the family home was run by the wife, it was the woman who carried on the daily offering of incense to the household god. The care of the tablets, the notation of the care of the ancestors, and cleaning the ancestral clan hall (a public room built to house the tablets) was also carried out by women.

The most important Confucian philosopher after "The Master" was Mang-tz (Mencius).[9-12] In his view, mankind was, by nature, good; social problems did not exist because of the nature of mankind, but as a result of the wickedness of government. Crime and disorder resulted from poverty and ignorance. Therefore Mencius recommended compulsory education for all.

According to written records, religious sacrifice existed and not only infants were put to death.[13,14] The oracular inscriptions found in the archaeological digs in China indicate that up through the Shang[15] period human sacrifice, primarily of enemies, was practiced. We have evidence that specific human sacrifices were made until at least 531 B.C. Prior to that time the practice was more extensive, though there was a developing cultural conscience against it.

In early ancient China during times of distress caused by droughts and famine, it was expected that the king or emperor might offer himself as a human sacrifice if necessary as a way to reverse the plight of his people.[16]

In the early history there was also an annual sacrifice to the river god during which a young girl was offered in marriage to the god. The girl would be placed on a bed that had been painted and bedecked with jewels. The bed was then placed in the river and floated about ten miles before it sank and the girl drowned.

During the Chou dynasty (1122-255 B.C.) there is evidence that different forms of human sacrifice were practiced.[17] A prisoner's throat might be cut and the blood smeared on the war drums prior to an attack. Or, upon return from a successful expedition, prisoners might be sacrificed to the ancestors or to the gods of the soil, their heads or ears buried before the entrance of the ancestral temple. If there was inadequate sun or rain in summer, a sorcerer might be put to death to appease the gods. Usually it was a female sorceress but occasionally a male sorcerer as well, or shaman. At times these sorcerers were required to dance in the sun until rain fell. This would sometimes continue to the point of death. Or, at their own request they would be buried alive with their heads exposed in the bright sunshine as an offering to the rain god. Sometimes hunchbacks or cripples would be tortured to appease the gods so that rain would come. All this ended with the Chou dynasty, though some such primitive practices continued in the rural areas.[18]

With this background of China's history and religious philosophy we turn to explore the family.[19-27] We will observe the expression of this history and philosophy in family life and its effects upon women and children. Of central importance was filial piety. Filial piety[28-30] required reverence for family and ancestry through service, offerings, and prayers. Face referred to a person's public moral and social standing. Inappropriate behavior, or failure at a public activity, could cause loss of face to oneself and one's family. Losing face was a great shame and embarrassment for the family.

The families lived in an extended network in small, rural communities, protected by walls. Neighbors left the walled villages to plant and cultivate crops, often assigning guards to protect their little communities while other villagers slept. What we find, then, is an interlocking pattern of human and natural existence—paradoxical among a people who were at once superstitious, but also skeptical, pious, pragmatic, and lacking any clerical or religious domination.

In pre-7th century B.C. China there were two classes, the patrician (including noblemen), and the commoner, with two distinct life-styles. While the patrician was free to talk, think, travel, and improve his lot, the commoner or the peasant lived simply in small restricted communities where the way of life was determined by the change of seasons—the indoor season and the outdoor. The season affected the common man's entire way of life, even his morals—easygoing and loose in summer, strict and formal in winter.

The Chinese favored large families, the ideal throughout their history. Since more than 90% of the Chinese farmed, large families were an advantage. Only during times of impoverishment (famine, flood, disaster) was infanticide practiced. The moral code of China made sexual relations an orderly process for raising a family and the primary reason for marriage. There could never be too many children.

Each family had one male leader who bore the family name—there were no personal names—and the entire family was obedient to him. He was in charge of marrying off sons and daughters and could dissolve marriages at will. If his finances permitted, he could marry more than one woman. In that case he would have a principal wife and secondary wives, all of whom had to come from the same clan. (The many families who could claim an honored important ancestor, and joined together in various enterprises were clans.) The secondary wives were subordinate (in running the home and general honors and respect) to the "first wife." The children were ranked according to the rank of their mother.

During the feudal period in China, despite the strict concept of filial piety, there was often conflict between sons and fathers. This happened because fathers were permitted to have sexual relations with women of their sons' generation and occasionally with their son's wife. Occasionally a son approached his father's concubines. This is one of the problems that Confucius tried to resolve in his teachings, which stressed that the rights of the individual should be safeguarded.

The Chinese father had power comparable to the *paterfamilias* of ancient Rome, with certain important differences. The *paterfamilias* owned all family property, while the Chinese father was considered only temporary custodian of the family property and could not bequeath the estate to a stranger or disinherit his sons at will. Property had to be divided equally among all sons. Aside from ancestor worship, marriage and family were one of the most important aspects of life in China.

In the typical home, the sexes were separated except at mealtime. The basis of all relationships centered around the father and son. Every other relationship was subordinate and supplementary to this basic relationship.

The wife's familial duty was to her husband, but even more to her husband's father. If there was a quarrel between a man's parents and his wife, the husband was expected to side with his parents. Realistically, there was little contact between father-in-law and daughter-in-law, and much more between the mother-in-law and the daughter-in-law.

Nonpatrician women[31-34] rose early, did hard physical labor, and retired early in the evening. The men, on the other hand, rose late, did moderate work, drank tea, and retired later than their wives and mothers. The women did laundry and the male made genealogical records, performed rituals, or propitiated the gods. In public, men exhibited their authority over their wives. In no quarrel could the wife triumph, because losing face meant losing money. A man who could not control his wife was considered a bad risk in business. Public knowledge of trouble at home could cause a man bankruptcy.

Though incest was forbidden, the ideal form of marriage

was between a father's sister's son and a mother's brother's daughter—unrelated cousins. The double marriage of two sisters from one family to two brothers of another family was also applauded.

The main responsibility in marriage was the propagation of the ancestral line. A woman's obligation was to produce sons and obey her husband and her parents-in-law. The remarriage of a widower was normal. A widow was expected to remain unmarried and mourn her dead husband. Male infidelity was common; female infidelity was social suicide.

A woman was judged for her sexual fidelity, sense of humility, and her ability to conform to three subordinations, to the father, husband, and son. Good behavior meant respect to husband, parents-in-law, living harmoniously with sisters-in-law, and observing the sexual taboo days.

The negative qualities that would weigh against men and women were indulgence in liquor, licentiousness, excess wealth, anger, violence, pride, hatred, jealousy, not studying the classics, criminality, running a gambling den, extravagance, gossiping, refusing to help those in need, and gluttony.

Only women were held accountable for licentiousness, disharmony, divorce, marriage against the mother's wishes, seduction, adultery, and running a brothel for profit rather than as a service to the community. Though murder was considered the most evil human deed, an unfaithful woman could be so severely punished she might die as a consequence.

To understand the concept of the clan family unit it is important to remember that the Chinese had a strong father/son identification, a cultural ideal to produce a large family, as well as a belief in the glorification of ancestors. Families within the clans shared wealth and glory for the clan's sake. These ideals were shaken during times of famine, when even the commoners felt forced to practice infanticide in order to survive.

Paradoxically, when a father succeeded in life, his son would not have to work hard. A man and his son might labor hard to earn money for the clan. The son, now prosperous, could indulge his own son by allowing him to be indolent as a mark of prestige—a system by which future generations suffered. By the fifth generation so much had been lost that the cycle of hard work would begin again.

A father could not abuse his power within the family without injuring himself, since the son was required to support and please his father and the father was required to provide for his son at all times. When the son married he remained under his father's supervision. As a son matured his father deferred to him more often. A son was expected to please his father and treat him fairly and lovingly. Independence was avoided. Since it was sensible not to do anything to disturb one's father, the son could not be considered fully mature as long as his father was alive.

Within the family unit money was shared. However, after a father divided his property among his sons, each household maintained its own finances. Borrowing between brothers was like borrowing from an outsider. There was keen competition between brothers and it was therefore not uncommon for them to dislike each other. Often the clans appeared unified but were divided internally. Though it was not always so, for the past 2000 years the head of the Chinese family has maintained his power essentially through love and respect rather than by any punitive measures. In fact, the greatest power was considered held by the one who taught the child the most. Thus a teacher could become the second and more significant father.

The ancient Chinese viewed their children as empty containers. They were the passive recipients of adult teachings and it was their duty to study, learn, and imitate. Their model, if not the parent, was the oldest male member of the household.

In poor families, though they learned basic skills of reading and writing, children were quickly directed toward physical labor, the kind necessary for family survival. These children learned by seeing and doing. They were reprimanded for their errors.

Instruction was not systematic. There were no classrooms and no particular theory.

Education,[35-38] if affordable, would prove important in later life. Chinese philosophy and government depreciated tradesmen and taxed them heavily. Still, there was extensive mercantile activity with countries both near and far. On a social scale, scholars were put at the highest level, followed by teachers, government officials, farmers, artisans, merchants, and, at the bottom of the scale, soldiers.

Though the civil service exams were open to all who wanted to take them (and anyone who worked for the government was part of this extensive civil service system), only those parents with at least a moderate income could provide their children with the education necessary to take even the preliminary exams.

China had an extensive civil service system for many centuries prior to Genghis Khan (13th century). Examinations were exceptionally difficult and required great proficiency. A person who passed the first level examination received a degree of Hsiu Ts'ai—the first literate class—and could be appointed to some minor local office. Those who wished could apply for further examination at the provincial level. If they passed the second test they were then eligible for appointment to minor positions in national service and were also admitted to the final and especially severe examinations in the capital of the country.

At the capital those tested would spend two or three days in an examination cell without any external support. Testing was rigorous and designed to determine knowledge of character and judgment, not knowledge of science, business, or industry.

With their lives of repression and deference to parental authority children's hostility would often show itself in some covert way. With the daughter-in-law subservient to the mother-in-law, and the secondary wives to the primary, repression was strong. When the daughter-in-law became a mother-in-law herself she might take out her hostility on her new daughter-in-law. Yet despite the difficulties and struggles within the family unit, family life flourished. Chinese dynasties lasted much longer along hereditary lines than did those of Europe. The only comparable dynasties were those of ancient Egypt.

The clan's punitive power[39-42] was approved by the central government as a logical extension of its normal moral authority. The central government maintained control over treason, murder, and major criminal offenses. Other offenses fell to the rule of the clan and the clan council.

The lord over the patrician was given absolute obedience. He operated within a strict and powerful feudal system that was even stronger than the filial piety. The one rule that controlled the overlord was that he was forbidden to fight a former teacher since the teacher had become a second father, thus taking preeminence over his biological father.

Government punished the guilty by flogging, chaining, banishing, enslaving, or imprisoning—any of which carried such a stigma, it was possible for the clan to banish them, as well, deeming the culprit a nonperson. The person without a clan, the nonperson, was in danger of starving. Without the clan there was no ready source of food or money.

The most common cause of clan punishment was filial impiety. Respect was to have been taught by the parents. Girls or boys guilty of impiety were not only responsible for the act, their parents were held responsible as well.

From ancient times the Chinese parent would prevent fighting among the children. Since filial impiety was such a blot on the clan, the clans would urge the father to exercise his powerful parental authority without abuse, and only for the family's well being. In fact, the government had written standards to which a family was expected to adhere: "A family in governing itself has four objectives. The first objective is education to raise the family social standing through the official careers of its members. The second objective is thrift so that the family can accumulate more wealth through saving. The third objective is harmony for the purpose of maintaining a well ordered domestic life. The last objective is to follow ethical teachings which keep the family from declining" (Tsung Standards).[43]

In general, mothers were more loving to their children than fathers. These roles were taught: the strict father, the kind and loving mother. In fact, the Chinese ideograph for kindness is a sign for mother and quite different than the ideograph for father, which is of a raised stick.

There were two main ages related to the Chinese family. First was the clan-dominated age, the feudal period (1100-250 B.C.). The second was the family-dominated age, the imperial period (250 B.C.-1900 A.D.). Since before the Ming and perhaps even prior to the Mongol period, the basic social unit of the traditional Chinese family has remained static. A 1926 study of China by a Western scholar made the interesting observation that "it is improbable that the Chinese have little added to, or more than superficially changed any of their fundamental social principles, since the compilation of the Ritual of Chou (12th century B.C.) and that of the Records of Rites (6th century B.C.)."

Clan domination diminished under the impact of non-Chinese ideas beginning in the Mongol period and further under Western ideas during the Ming restoration. This led to an increase in family domination and a decline in the prevalence of the extended family.

In the extended family, or clan, a young member who broke the rules was first warned by the head of the clan. If the offender did not reform he would be beaten by the head of the clan. If he continued defiant the government authorities would be asked to banish the offender to a distant place, making him a nonperson. Rarely would the head of a clan request that a culprit be put to death and then only under extreme conditions. But if a parent committed suicide because of a child's behavior, the child was held responsible and put to death.

Among the ancient Chinese there were generally two philosophical positions: adhering to a rigid code of law, or following custom. *Li* was the complex of customs and *Fa* was the positive written law. As is customary in China, the two factions compromised, this time by setting cultural legal standards.

When it came to civil issues, Li was the rule that was followed. When it came to criminal issues, Fa, a much more rigid standard, was followed. In China, spiritual moral values were much more important than the law. Chinese law became essentially an administrative act, when moral (family/clan) pressure did not succeed or did not apply. The oldest recorded code of law was written in 535 B.C. These laws had a strong moral flavor, and were based on earlier rules of conduct.

The spirit of Li was to "prevent guilt being fixed on the innocent." There was even a requirement in Chinese law that all cases where the death sentence had been pronounced must be reviewed. Human life was precious in China, despite evidence of aberrations such as infanticide and child slavery.

In China, crime was considered a disturbance in the order of nature which had to be rectified. Thus, the 7th century B.C. Chou Code stated: "It is dangerous and ominous to leave Li and engage in legally fixed punishments." According to Chinese law, it was not rights that were guaranteed. Rather it was duties and mutual compromises governed by order, responsibility, hierarchy, and harmony in all things that had to be preserved. The goal was to demonstrate justice and organic unity.

As noted earlier, a punishment that came from outside the clan was seen as a stigma. Though there was great emphasis upon the law, it was a framework for people to look to if not actually utilize. In some sizable towns years could pass without any case coming to court.

Though the laws were codified under the Chou dynasty they dealt primarily with crime and not with civil matters. Trials were simple with no lawyers needed to argue for either side. A judge (a person of high repute and power) examined all the issues and came to a conclusion. His examination was presented in public before the jury, sometimes the entire town. When he came to a conclusion and pronounced punishment on the criminal, the town would usually support him. However, if the people decided he erred in judgment, it was the judge who then had to accept the punishment. Historically there is little evidence of any corruption in the courts.

It is understandable then that a judge might verbally denounce the convicted person, but the actual physical punishment usually would be minimal in case an error had been made. The judge not only protected himself but protected the community, for all court proceedings were public and the people would agree with the judge's disapproval, which was very controlling on the miscreant.

Though punishments were sometimes severe, they were never as severe or as cruel in China as in Western civilization. Punishment ranged from cutting off hair and flogging, to banishment and death. If the criminal was of a very high rank he was given the option of committing suicide and there were often generous commutations of sentences. In normal periods only the emperor could inflict capital punishment. However, if he ruled unjustly by common consent he would lose the "mandate of heaven" and could be deposed without breaking any moral or legal law.

The great unifier of China, Ch'in Shih-huang, tried to establish an extensive legalistic state based on the writings of Shang Yng. He established a book of rules of the ruler of Shan (Shang-chun-Chou).[44] This book has influenced the legal system in China ever since the 4th century B.C. There was a return to Confucianism after the Chin period, based on the concept that man had an infinite capacity to perfect himself, through continued study of himself and ancient traditions. Chinese law is essentially Confucianist in its origin, the ideal character being summed up in the term *Chutzu*. This ideal person would recognize injustice in the state and do everything within his power to combat it.

Until Western thought was introduced into China, the Chinese never saw any need to issue a separate set of codes for civil and criminal law. They believed that it was the primary responsibility of the community and family to deter, detect, prevent, and prosecute any offense that took place within its confines.

Shame became a fundamental element of control. The book *The Principle of Harmony* (Zhou Li) states that shame should be used in controlling the individual in the community. The criminal must be reeducated and saved from himself. The person who is supposed to reeducate the criminal is called the rescuer. His function is to take charge of people who exhibit evil "or depraved propensities, or commits acts of error; to rebuke and punish them; and to rescue them by restraining them with preventive proprieties." After a man was rebuked three times he would be flogged. After having been flogged three times, if he continued unregenerate he would be sent to a judge who would have fastened to his back a tablet bearing descriptions of his offense. He would have his person exposed to shame on the Good Rock (*Jishi*). After this he would be put to labor under the minister of works (relative slavery). When they were returned to their communities the convicted criminals would not, for three years, be accorded the privileges and seniority to which their age might entitle them. But if they behaved correctly they would once more be accepted by the community.

The clan unit "law" can be summed up by the basic philosophy of Zhougong: respect for virtue; respect for age; those in high places giving to those in lower echelons; those who succeed giving to those who fall; advancement through self-improvement; and moderation in all things through self-discipline.

The "Ten Commandments" that are part of ancestral worship and the mourning process gives us further understanding of the Chinese sociopsychological legal construction:

1. Thou shalt not forget about filial piety and harmony among brothers.
2. Thou shalt not violate the law of the nation and offend and cheat the ruler.
3. Thou shalt not forget about the dignity of teachers or show signs of ingratitude.
4. Thou shalt not disrupt relations within the lineage and clan.
5. Thou shalt not fight or seek revenge so as to disturb the village and the neighborhood.
6. Thou shalt not refuse to come to the rescue of those who are urgently in need.
7. Thou shalt not cheat and be unaware of the necessity in accumulating spiritual goods.
8. Thou shalt not take advantage of special positions and privileges and cause inconvenience to others.
9. Thou shalt not expose other peoples' secrets.
10. Thou shalt not disobey any commandments.

The commandments did not apply to small children or those who were unaware of them or unable to understand them.

The Book of Laws[45] contains some 2900 pages. Following are excerpts which pertain to families and children:

1. Aged and infirm were not to be tried, even if at the time of offense they might not have been in such a classification. (This indicates a special awareness of, care for, and protection of the weak and helpless, therefore, less child abuse.)

2. Youth had privileges, when the age of the offender at the time of the crime did not exceed 15 years, no matter the age at the subsequent trial. (This shows an understanding of differences in capabilities and the nonmature state of the adolescent as well as of the child.)

3. "Whoever receives and detains the strayed or lost child of a free person, and instead of presenting to the magistrate,

sells such a child as a slave, shall be punished with 100 blows, and three years banishment. Whoever sells such a child for marriage or adoption to any family, shall be punished with 90 blows and banishment for 2½ years. Whoever so disposes of a strayed or lost slave shall suffer the punishment provided by this law." (Clearly this indicates that the kind of abuse of children that occurred in Greece and Rome was far less likely to occur in China.)

4. A husband could repudiate his wife if she gave him one of the seven justifying causes for a divorce. However, those did not apply if she did one of the three following things: "(1) Mourned for three years her husband's parents; (2) if the family was poor when they started and now had become rich; and (3) the wife had no living parents to receive her back again." (The protection of women and the limitation of the man's power over her is clear. Though the female was inferior to the male, she had rights and protection recognized by the community.)

5. The law prevented any family from having its property or freedom taken away, except in cases of treason. (This law clearly limits the power of authority, such as of nobles, etc.— something quite rare in the West.)

6. The power of the son/father filial piety relationship was stressed by laws that punished a son if he did not properly mourn for his deceased parent. In fact, he could not even absent himself to hold a governmental position if there was not proper care provided by other adult members of the family for his parents and grandparents. (The law demonstrates how central the family was and how the government supported that position.)

7. A husband could beat or even kill his wife if she were discovered in the act of adultery. However, if a husband did not immediately punish his wife, but delayed it, then he would not be permitted to punish her himself but would have to go to clan or court jurisdiction. "If a wife commits a crime within the family unit but not one worthy of death, and the husband kills her, he shall suffer the punishment of death by being strangled."

(Here is a clear expression of the inferiority of women and the power of a husband over her, but with some limitations. It does stress family intactness, with a one-sided view.)

8. One activity that required a death sentence that was intrafamilial was the striking of a parent or grandparent. Parents, on the other hand, could not punish their children severely, for if the child was injured or died, the parent would be punished with 100 blows or even put to death. (Thus, though an older child could be punished, it would not apply if the parents were at fault.)

9. Infanticide was illegal for 2000 years in China's history. (This law indicates a community/government attitude that only broke down when government broke down [e.g., warring states, conquest] or families broke down, as in times of plague, famine, or flood.)

10. No relative or child could be punished by the court unless the relatives who were offended, including the parents, directly complained. The complaint could not come from an outsider. (This clearly shows how the government wished to stay out of family [also clan] problems. Only if the family was nonfunctional could the "law" apply.)

11. Intercourse with a female under 12 years of age was considered rape, and in all cases rape was punished by at least 100 blows. Anyone forcing a child female member of their household to engage in criminal intercourse would be punished with at least 100 blows. There were also many instances where the rapist would be beheaded. (The protection of the most vulnerable part of society [the female child or servant] is evident here.)

12. "It shall not, in any tribunal or government, be permitted to put to question by torture those who belong to any of the eight privileged classes, in consideration due to the respect of their character; to those who have obtained their 70th year, in consideration to their grand state; to those who have not acceded to their 15th year, out of indulgence to their tender youth;

and lastly to those who labor under any permanent disease or infirmity, out of commiseration for their situation and sufferings." (Again, we see the protection of the weak and helpless.)

13. "Moreover—in the case of individuals who are 80 or under ten years of age or are entirely and permanently infirm, it shall not be permitted even to require or to receive their testimony, even without torture." (This indicates that it was understood by all that the very young and the very old may not perceive their world accurately.)

14. "Female offenders shall not be committed to prison except in capital cases, or cases of adultery. In all other cases, they shall, if married, remain in the charge and custody of their husbands, and if single, in their relations or next neighbors, who shall, upon every such occasions, be responsible for their appearance in a tribunal of justice, when required." It was also found that no woman could be questioned, interrogated, or imprisoned if she were pregnant, and until 100 days had elapsed from the time of her delivery. (The extra protection for women [more than men] and the involvement of family is a vital point.)

15. Any attempt, successful or not, homosexually to rape a boy under 12 years of age was cause for death. (The more severe penalty for homosexual rape of a male child indicates that the Chinese felt homosexuality of males was unacceptable, abuse of a child unacceptable, and that abusing a boy was worse than abusing a girl.)

The laws were enforced extensively, especially among the middle and patrician class. As we have seen, they paid special attention to women and children in a very protective way. Let us look more closely at the status of women in this society.

Though single women of nobility were very restricted, married woman were much freer, and there was ample opportunity for them to have sexual affairs in and out of the home. This was true from 700 B.C. until the Confucian ethics took hold. It was also during this period that some sons were permitted to have sexual relations with their father's wives, excluding their own mother. The difference between the nobility and the common people was that the nobility restricted sexual activity only before marriage while the common people restricted sexual activity only after marriage.

Marriage[46-52] in China had little to do with love. Its main purpose was to bring healthy mates together so they could rear abundant families. Most marriages were arranged by parents. Celibacy in marriage was a crime against the ancestors and the state, and there were officials who saw to it that celibacy was not practiced. Neighbors spied on neighbors and the offender was subjected to extended interrogation.

Polygamy was acceptable for respectable men if they could afford more than one wife. Sometimes the primary wife would employ concubines for her husband or would arrange for a second or third wife. The first wife would be the most important and would have the most power in the home.

There were six rites leading up to marriage: (1) inquiries made of the girl's family by an intermediary; (2) genealogical and horoscopic data about the bride was collected; (3) the girl's horoscope was matched with the boy's; (4) the betrothal was sanctified by a transfer of gifts; (5) the date of the wedding was fixed; and (6) the bride was married and physically moved to the household of her new husband.

Before a man married he had no property rights in his family or clan. After he married he had rights equal to any other married male in the family unit. Though the girl's family gave up rights to their daughter when they transferred her to her husband's family, they retained an interest in her well being. Though a woman could be divorced by her husband for almost any reason, she could not divorce her husband. She might leave him, however, though that would be a grave insult, and return to her parents' home. It was a clan decision if any property was to be returned with her.

When a woman became pregnant, she was expected to abstain from violent emotion, from eating certain foods, and from looking at "terrible things." She was responsible for the education of the fetus. Her behavior was thought to affect the future personality of the child. The father, meanwhile, was only expected to abstain from sexual relations with his wife, as this might affect the physiological development of the child and might lead to its early death. Since fear could cause tension in the household, the pregnant woman was relieved of household chores that might cause her any anxiety or unhappiness. For a month prior to and a month after delivery, women were confined. They were not permitted to pass through the main entrance of the family home. Their bodies were thought unclean and might give offense to the gods who were guarding the entrance.

Just before the child was delivered, a special medicinal soup was fed to the mother by her parents. Thus we can see that a girl who left her family home when she married maintained a relationship with her parents. In fact, upon delivery it was her mother, rather than her mother-in-law's responsibility to look after the daughter's clothes and to wait on her. She moved into the daughter's home to do this and returned to her own after about one week.

Until the Ching (Manchu) dynasty (1644-1912) there was no prudery in China about the important sexual matters of life. Prior to that dynasty there were a series of handbooks about sex that were considered manuals for teaching the householder (men and women) how to conduct sexual relations. These books were studied by Chinese people for 2000 or more years— especially until the 13th century A.D. The invasion of the Mongols under Genghis Khan made this study a more private affair inside the home, as the Chinese withdrew more into their sequestered world.

According to Taoism women were credited with having a particularly strong *te*, or quality of virtue. This could be given to a man, since a woman had the power to bind a man to her—not by her beauty, but by her feminine magic. Not only did a woman have *te*, but, jade had it too, and could therefore be used to preserve people.

In this very early ancient culture[53-56] (pre-Chin 250 B.C.) wives were buried alive when their husbands died if the husbands were important public figures. The wife's *te* was used to preserve the husband in the afterlife. Also, upon their death, emperors were often buried with their wives, concubines, or slaves. When Ch'in Shih-huang died around 280 B.C., several hundred maidens were buried alive to keep him company. The workmen who brought the coffin into the tomb were buried alive so that they would not reveal the secret passage into the grave. This is the last known time that people were buried alive or killed when an emperor died. Of 86 tombs excavated at Hsun Hsien, only one case was found where there may have been human sacrifice. This practice was completely stopped by 100 B.C., and instead of slaves (to serve them in the afterlife) or wives and others being buried alive or killed, effigies were used instead. Swords and armor and other articles, including horses and chariots, were buried with models of soldiers and servants. In much later ages, paper models of the dead man's house were burned as an offering, a practice that continued until recent times as a remnant of this ancient Chou custom.

Since royalty had more *te* than the commoner, it was believed that royal Chinese were able to worship their ancestors better. The nobility protected the power of the woman's *te* and often kept women separate to make sure virgin women would be married without having given up their *te*. The common people had no such practice nor did they have as much *te*. As a result, there was a great deal more freedom for their women, sexually and otherwise, before marriage.

The union of kings and queens was considered the *sine qua non* for harmony in the land. The Chinese believed that natural disasters were caused by poor sexual relations between the ruler and his spouse. The sexual activity of the king and queen was carefully regulated by various rites. Because the king had more need for *te* than anyone, he needed a large number of females with *te* to supply him through repeated sexual intercourse. Thus he had a large number of queens, consorts, wives of first, second, and third rank, and concubines. The ranking was determined by social class, family power, political expediency, and royal fiat. Court ladies (*nu-shih*) had the responsibility of regulating and supervising the sexual relations of the king and his many wives. The *nu-shih* would conduct the women to the royal bedchamber and would watch to make sure consummation had occurred. Only the highest rank of wives or consorts could spend the entire night with the king.

With Taoism reigning in the home, naturalism or a natural response to sexual matters was the common rule. Following the Mongol invasion, a more puritanical, Confucianist attitude reigned. An understanding of the authentic Chinese attitude toward sex is more accurate if practices are viewed prior to the Mongol period. Until the 13th century sexual relations were freely written about and talked about, though not in a pornographic sense. The West's understanding of Chinese (social and sexual) habits until the Ching period was based mostly on the distorted writings of Marco Polo, whose contacts were principally with Mongols and Turks.

It seems that prior to the 13th century A.D., women were always considered sexually superior to men. Women were supposed to have special magical powers, particularly in sexual matters. This open attitude toward sex changed after the Mongol conquest, when the Han withdrew to their private world.

The Chinese handbooks[57,58] always represented the female as the guardian of the knowledge of sex. The woman was the initiator of sex, and the man was her ignorant pupil. Even with the prevalence of the patriarchal system, when it came to sexual matters, it was the responsibility of the woman to teach her husband on the wedding night. Woman is called the "great mother" who nourishes not only her offspring but also her husband and who, during the sexual act, "feeds and strengthens his limited life source by tapping into her inexhaustible supply." The ideograph for marriage shows the relationship of husband and wife as the character *ch'i*, where the woman is on the same level as the man. The history of the ideograph indicates that the husband and wife would respect each other as guests in the same dwelling. Thus the basic construction of the relationship in the family unit was, by these ancient standards, thought to be equal, with the man dominant outside of the household and the woman dominant within it. This meant that everything involving the care of children, cooking, washing, maintaining the home, and directing servants, was under the wife's control.

In ancient China, the original shamans (similar to witch doctors) were female, and only later did the shaman become a male. In its earliest times China was a matriarchy, typical of an agricultural society. In fact, in the ancient magical rites the deity of drought and the deity of rain were both goddesses.[59]

Later, the power of women waned and matriarchy was replaced by a clan-operated partial patriarchy. The status of women became inferior, particularly among the patricians. Among the common people women were not as segregated as elsewhere in the world, nor were they considered intrinsically inferior to men. Material related to the Yin/Yang of Taoism, and the necessity for developing a family line based on males all contributed to maintaining and respecting the vital role of the woman. Her sexuality and ability to produce strong healthy children meant having girls as well as boys, for that was the only way the clan could continue. Though a girl would eventually leave her immediate family, she would still marry within the clan and maintain the clan's strength. Women were absolutely necessary to maintain the sanctity of family lineage and uphold the honor of the clan. The ancient maxim ran: "A son is honored because of his mother; and a mother is honored because of her son." Though women were honored, they were of lower status than men.

The official marriage ceremony included these words: "Welcome your mate to carry on your bloodline. Later by mutual respect she is to be the heir and successor to your own mother, to your own grandmother. Respect your mate even as you respect your mother, your grandmother." During the marriage ceremony the groom was expected to symbolize his readiness to serve his bride in every way, even as a servant. Most Chinese practiced monogamy, though polygamy was practiced among the very wealthy. We find that the incidence of wife beating in China is rare. In fact, the translation of a word related to "wife" is "she who must be obeyed." Wife beating was a punishable offense.

Though there was public disapproval of romantic love, there was extensive training for it. A man usually came to a marriage unprepared to fully understand sexuality. His wife, however, had been so trained. She had studied sexuality from a book and would teach her husband after they were married. This was a change from the earlier Tang period, when there was greater freedom between the sexes.

In the later Chou dynasty (500 B.C.) there was extreme social disturbance—wars, feudalism—and a slackening of morals among the nobility. Noblemen began keeping harems for entertainment, and girls were used in a variety of sexual activities with their master, his retinue, and his guests. Also, some of the young princes began keeping boys as catamites—boys used for anal sex (*luan-tung*).

The normal sexual activity between a man and woman was seen as part of cosmic nature: the clouds were the ovum, the rain was the emission of semen from man. The reverse of clouds and inverted rain was the ideographic depiction of homosexuality. Thus homosexuality was always considered abnormal and not part of the natural cosmic order.

The Confucianist school, which arose as a means of controlling anarchy, brought puritanism to the life of the people. Part of their activity was establishing male superiority and treating women as inferior to men (the opposite of Taoism).

In the pre-Han period the Chinese had the following ideas

about sex: (1) no clear concept of physiological functions of female generative activity. All the secretions and fluids of the uterus and vagina had a Yin essence (*te*). Man's semen was limited in quantity, but a woman had an inexhaustible supply of Yin. (2) Intercourse had two purposes, to have a woman conceive and to strengthen a man's vitality by his absorbing some of the woman's Yin essence. (3) A woman could become healthier by a stirring of her latent Yin nature. (4) To conceive healthy male children, the male's Yang essence had to be at its apex when he ejaculated. To achieve this he had to have sexual relations with different women without ejaculating and then, when his Yang reached its apex, he would have sexual relations with his primary wife when her Yin was at its apex. (5) A man should give the woman complete satisfaction every time he had sex with her and have it frequently so she would have increased Yin essence. Thus, masturbation for a man was forbidden, but encouraged for a woman. (6) Since a man had to retain as much of his essence as possible he would train himself to have retrograde ejaculation. (7) Men had to learn to prolong coitus without reaching an orgasm. The longer he was able to have intercourse, the more Yin essence would be stimulated in the woman and absorbed by him, thus strengthening his vital force.

Male homosexuality was frowned on, since there was a danger of losing male essence; but female homosexuality was encouraged, since there was no genital union and the stimulation would increase the Yin essence. Lesbianism could only occur within the female quarters of a home and was praised because it increased the harmony within the home. In addition to the obvious techniques of finger and tongue there was also a double olisbos (a short stick made of wood or ivory that had two silk bands attached to the middle that would be tied to one woman and then used as a penis). Another object that was primarily for masturbation was the exertion bell (*mien-ling*)—a small hollow ball of silver that was placed in the vagina prior to coitus. It also could be placed there for masturbation purposes.

Female homosexuality was widespread in China and male homosexuality was quite rare until the Han dynasty. During the Han dynasty homosexuality by males was occasionally seen as fashionable and it reappeared during the Northern Sung dynasty (960-1127 A.D.). From that time to the Ching dynasty (1644 A.D.), male homosexuality was less common in China than anywhere else. In fact, in 111 A.D. a law was written that prescribed that any man caught engaging in homosexual activities should be struck 100 times with a bamboo cane.

The handbooks of the art of sexuality contained explicit instructions on how a man should prepare a woman for sexual union. All the foreplay and the variety of positions were described in a serious manner, not for entertainment. The purpose of the variety was to maintain the man's interest in his conjugal responsibilities and duties. For example, fellatio was permitted but never to reach a climax, while cunnilingus was approved because it prepared the woman for the act and also gave the man some of the Yin essence from the woman.

Sexual relations with prostitutes were considered completely separate from sexual activity in the home. Prostitutes were recreational, while the sexual activity in the home was for the purpose of producing children, particularly male heirs. The taboos on what could or could not be done sexually with one's wife were lifted in sexual relations with a prostitute.

In the Chinese texts describing proper sexual activity a section about prenatal care and diet was included. Procreation was a part of the order of nature and a sacred duty of every man and woman.

In the history of China we see that Taoists considered women more equal to men than Confucians. Confucius considered women inferior to men but he did not despise them. Throughout their history, then, the Chinese never came close to depreciating women to the degree that the early Romans and Greeks did. And the Chinese never viewed sex as a sin. In fact, one of the most important rights for a woman, more than for a man, was the right to sexual satisfaction. Texts on this subject (*L-Chi*) refer to sexual neglect of a woman as a grave offense. *L-Chi* specifically states that neither age nor beauty should make a husband deviate from the strict protocol, set procedures, and frequency of sexual intercourse with his wives and concubines. "Even if a concubine is growing older, as long as she has not yet reached the age of 50, the husband shall copulate with her every five days. She on her part shall, when she is led to his couch, be cleanly washed, neatly attired, have her hair combed and properly done up, and wear a long robe and properly fastened house shoes." These conjugal duties ceased when he became 70.

During the Han dynasty there were strict regulations about the separation of men and women to maintain the proper moral climate. This indicated that there had been moral laxity prior to the Han. Some evidence of this is seen in the history of Emperor Hsiao-Ching (156-140 B.C.), whose relatives were considered degenerates and sadists because they had sexual relations with their sisters.

The Han emperors tried to bring order into the empire, primarily to the royal house, by demonstrating appropriate sexual activity. In public, they practiced the Confucianist attitude of propriety, but behind the bedroom doors the orgies continued. Homosexuality was practiced among the royalty, but there is no evidence of sexual activity with children.

In the later Han dynasty foreign trade expanded, the middle class grew, and the demand for houses of prostitution increased as more travelers and merchants visited China. Although acceptable for the middle class, it was considered improper for an educated man to go to a brothel. With a larger middle class, this activity increased and changed the tone of city life. It was during the later Han that the books on the *Art of the Bedchamber* were formalized into a series of texts forming eight volumes. They were illustrated and were part of every bride's trousseau. She was required to study these texts to teach her sexually innocent husband.

According to the *Art of the Bedchamber*,[60] "Woman is superior to man in the same respect as water is superior to fire. Those who are expert in sexual intercourse are like good cooks who know how to blend the five flavors into tasty broth." For the sexual act to be appropriate, a man and woman were to be in harmony. It was to be avoided when a man was intoxicated, after a heavy meal, or if he was upset in any way. The text also warned that a man must never force himself on a woman in a sexual act, and that the woman must reach an orgasm during every sexual act.

What is notably missing from all Chinese literature, particularly the *Art of the Bedchamber*, is material about sexual perversions.[61] Though Chinese histories refer to various forms of cruelty, there is no indication of sexual satisfaction related to it—no material on sadomasochism.

Bestiality was unknown in Chinese literature, although incest was common in the courts in the Chu kingdom and the former Han court. It later became quite rare. In fact it was classified in the penal code as an inhuman act to be punished by death. Some pornographic (scatological) material of limited nature is only found in the erotic novels of the later Ming period (17th century A.D.).[62,63]

The Tang dynasty (618-907 A.D.) established much of the cultural flavor that we know as Chinese. Its capital, Ch'ang-An (modern Sian), had a district where women were available for sexual pleasure. Once the women were inside this special quarter, they were automatically registered to enter and remain in any of the many walled compounds where they lived out their lives. They were rigorously trained in various skills and their "adopted mothers" would often whip them if they did not learn well. Their only chance to escape was if a guest would buy them and take them as a wife or concubine. These women tried to live up to the high standards set by the scholars who frequented their establishment. During this period scholars did frequent brothels; it was not accepted during the Han dynasty. Thus the courtesan became an important social institution in the capital and the main cities of the provinces. When a man traveled he left his various wives and concubines at home and took a courtesan with him for entertainment. It was also during this dynasty and on through the Ming period that excess drinking at banquets by both men and women became acceptable.

By the Mongol period prostitution had become a well organized trade. Brothel keepers united in trade associations and paid taxes directly to the government. Two levels of prostitution emerged from this system: the courtesan, who was highly placed in society, and the low-class harlots. To some men, one of the advantages of staying with a courtesan was that he wasn't required to have sexual relations with her. This was a welcome relief from his marital obligations at home.

During the Ming restoration,[64] which began in the 14th century A.D., the practice of purchasing concubines and lower class wives increased, and female virginity became rare. Divorce was now much more difficult. The texts describing proper marital sexual activity were less frequently circulated and there was more puritanism in the culture.

From a Western point of view, the widespread and ancient practice of footbinding[65-67] was an indication of how the Chinese demeaned women. Certainly, it was a painful and crippling process.

The practice began during the 10th century, when palace dancers bound their feet. At first the compression was only temporary and slight, and did not severely hamper movement. Much later, a woman who had been hobbled by this process had to lean on a cane for support. This occurred primarily among the upper classes. Large feet were considered grotesque and low-class. If a woman did not have her feet bound she was classified as a maid or slave girl and would not be eligible for any reasonable marriage.

Foot-binding reached its heights at the close of the Ming dynasty. This practice was minimal prior to the Mongol invasion and was essentially restricted to concubines, palace dancers, and entertainers. Following the Mongol invasion more Chinese women bound their feet, and the practice increased markedly by the 19th century. In fact, five volumes were written by Yao Ling Hsi on the subject.

The small-footed female has always been appealing to the Chinese male—the result of a national foot fetish that existed long before foot-binding became extensive. When foot-binding was condemned by the Chinese themselves, it was condemned on the basis of it being rude, lascivious, and overtly sexual. "It could lead a man astray and prevent him from fulfilling his social responsibilities." The Chinese compared their foot-binding practice to the Western practice of severe corseting, the popular "hourglass figure."

The bound female foot was given the name of "lotus," and foot lovers would adore being touched by it, especially as a prelude to the sexual act of coitus. Not only was the appearance and the touch important, but also the aroma that came from the bound foot as it was released from its bindings. Kissing, sucking the foot, putting the whole foot in the mouth, nibbling at it, chewing at it, having it pressed against the genitals, all were part of the sexual foreplay of the educated Chinese male.

Though foot-binding was a feminine monopoly, there were some instances of males binding their feet to achieve similar effects. Though this was essentially a Chinese practice, there is evidence that the Korean women tried to follow this procedure. The Manchu women, in defiance of official decree, as well as all upper-class Korean women during the Manchu period, practiced a form of footbinding in imitation of the upper-class Chinese woman whom they admired.

There were contests yearly in various provinces known as the "assemblage of foot viewing" and this continued into the Manchu dynasty. They also had "Tiny Foot Festivals." During one such festival, as reported by a Japanese student of the phenomenon, a woman who was older than 60 won first prize among 500 participants because her feet were less than three inches long. Some of the wealthier families dyed the woman's feet red since this would add to their beauty.

The distorted foot had a swollen ankle that was concealed by leggings with a diminutive foot toe encased in a very delicate boot; the leggings covered most of the boot except for the tip. The shoe, leggings, and boot were fashioned of silk, decorated with embroidery, and were very expensive.

Whenever the woman had sexual relations (with maidservants attending and assisting during the sexual activity) the shoes and leggings would remain on even though the rest of the woman's body would be naked. Only inside a special curtained bed and only for her husband, would a woman remove the leggings and shoes. The bandages about her feet would only be removed when she took a bath and exchanged her old leggings for fresh bandages.

There is no doubt that there were detrimental physical effects on the woman's health caused by foot-binding. However, if the child survived the footbinding, no secondary difficulties were likely to follow other than restriction on certain fast-moving physical activities, such as dancing, fencing, and physical exercise. These activities all were very popular with women prior to the foot-binding era.

It is interesting to note that during the Mongol conquest foot-binding became more popular and can be connected to an increased isolation of women in the home. Foot-binding was favored by the Confucian philosophers of the Mongol and Ming periods.

Slavery, too, was representative of the demeaned Chinese woman, for it was usually the daughter of a poor family who was sold into slavery during ancient times. Still, in early ancient China slavery was not a major factor in the economic or social structure of the culture. Those slaves who did exist were primarily used for domestic work, the salt and iron mines, and only occasionally in agriculture. Most domestic slaves were daughters of poor peasant families and were sold by their parents.

During Shang times (1766 B.C.),[68] the majority of slaves were used in royal households. Others, captives of foreign war, were used for human sacrifice in religious rituals. Domestic female servants (slave girls) were rarely used as human sacrifices. Sometimes the domestic slaves would be sacrificed at the death of their lord including some males who wore special hair braids indicating they were of socially inferior status ("barbarian"). The largest single category of slaves was the Ch'iang, a non-Chinese people of southwestern Shansi (probably Tibetan).

During the time of Confucius slavery was very minimal. Slaves were mostly used as servants in the few palaces. Slave girls were at the mercy of their mistresses, and even the children of the household sometimes beat them for sport. If they ran away they could not survive because they would be unable to understand or cope with the world around them. Often, they were picked up and sold into brothels. Many of these slave girls were sold when they were young. They were illiterate, ignorant, and unsophisticated and could not conceive of going to the authorities for help if they were abused. The authorities at this time did not consider this form of slavery other than benign.

It should be noted that in the Han[69] society of 202 A.D. slaves were never more than 1% of the population. Originally these were the male and female relatives of convicted criminals who had been confiscated by the government along with their other goods. Slaves were forced to obey the commands of their masters and were considered property. But the slave owners' rights were by no means unlimited and did not include the arbitrary power of life and death.

Slaves by and large did household and menial tasks. Sometimes they performed personal and special tasks including guard duty. During the Han period there were more slaves in the empire than at any other time, with the exception of more recent history—up until about 300 or 400 years ago—when slavery began to flourish in China. In fact, as recently as 1935 there were between two and four million child slaves in China.[70-77]

Now let us look closer at how this interplay of society, family, and women affected the lives of their children.[78-83]

Children normally were kept in the women's quarters of the house (except for the poorest peasant, who lived in 1 or 2 rooms) until the age of seven. At that age the children were separated. The boys went with their fathers and the girls continued to stay with their mothers. Chastity was not required of single males but was required of single females. Masturbation was encouraged for all females and was restricted for males.

In the earlier primitive periods in China among the patrician families, the birth of a boy was signaled with a mulberry branch. The branch was hung on the left side of the gate for a boy, and a napkin was hung on the right side of the gate for a girl. In general, as has been noted, mothers were more loving toward their children than fathers. These roles were taught— the strict father, the kind and loving mother. In fact, the Chinese ideograph for kindness is a sign for mother and is quite different from the ideograph for father, which is a raised stick.

Then, for the first three days of its life, the child would be left unfed and alone in a closed chamber—a boy on a bed, a girl on the floor. After three days the head of the family would decide whether to accept the child as part of the family or reject it, depending on the child's vitality. Those rejected were killed or exposed. Those accepted were taken by a servant who had been purified by fasting the same three days, and were carried to the mother's apartment where the mother or the wet nurse suckled it for the first time. The wet nurse was often a second wife if the first wife was unable to suckle the child.

In a rite for the male child, the head of the house would fashion a bow from the symbolic mulberry stick, make six arrows from grass stalks and would shoot them toward the sky, the earth, and each of the four directions to ward off potential calamities. For a female child the father announced that the family would make a sacrifice and keep the girl.

This marked the beginning of a three month period during which the child was still not fully accepted and was hidden in a separate room where its mother had to live apart from her husband and the other women until the three-month ceremony was completed. If the child was still vigorous it could be presented to the entire family—particularly to the father. The child was now accepted by his right hand and given a name, which the father would say in a falsetto, childish voice as not to frighten it.

In contrast, common men would accept all children born into the clan. They would need them to help work the fields. The life of the patrician child was different.

Unfortunately, the rate of infant and maternal mortality was high—caused by "evil spirits." The ancient Chinese held a ceremony (*manyu*) one month after a child was born at which a child would be bathed and given a personal name by its maternal uncle. This name had negative connotations—dog, cat, or monkey—but because it was negative the evil spirits would ignore the child. It was also believed that any outward show of affection for the child might cause the evil spirits to look at the child with favor. The parents would, therefore, avoid showing any outward expression of love to their children.

All infants were breast-fed. If the mother had no milk, porridge or cow's milk would be administered or, if there was a secondary wife or concubine who had milk, she might be a wet nurse. This was uncommon except among the very wealthy, where there might be three or four wives and many concubines. Diapering was exclusively by the women. After each diaper change the infant's lower body was rinsed with water, but there was no regular bathing.

An infant was never left unattended by the mother or some other woman in the household. All women in the household were extended mother surrogates. Occasionally a man would sit with the child after it was two or three months of age. He would hold it, give it food, caress it, even try to play with it, though he would never change its diapers. If the mother left home the infant would be tied to her with the child's stomach against her back. A male child would be carried this way longer than a female child, up to the age of three.

Toilet training began at 12 months. The mother held the child's back against her own abdomen, and lifted the child's legs to induce urination and defecation. She did not punish the child who was just learning, though a child who had not been trained by age 3 or 4 might be chastised. In general there was very little systematic training or enforcement of toilet training or dietary habits among the ancient Chinese.

Children would eat with adults as soon as they were able, and would eat whatever the adults were eating. Weaning occurred late. Children demanded adult food rather than being forced to eat.

In the less affluent homes children would sleep with their parents in the same room, sometimes the same bed, until they were 7 or 8 years of age, regardless of their sex. As a result, they learned the basic facts of sex by direct observation, though they were prohibited from showing curiosity about the genitals of the opposite sex.

In training a child, the most important consideration was to avoid deviating from the group morality and ethic. Individual comfort was of little concern; the point was to conform to the group. Historically, Chinese orientation toward children was essentially moralistic, not psychological. Adults were primarily concerned with control, discipline, and conformity, a philosophy that continues to this day.

In ancient times it was believed that if a child became ill, evil spirits were to blame. If the child died before 12 months, no ceremony took place. The body was simply taken out of the household, rolled in a straw mat and buried in some unused ground outside the town area. Usually wild dogs or swine would search it out and eat it. A wealthy family might attempt to avoid this by using some type of coffin. If more than one child died in close succession, the procedure was different. The face of the second child who died would be slapped by shoes, and its body would be thrown into a lake instead of being buried in the ground. It was thought that a life-stealing ghost (Tao Sa Guer) had intervened in the family's activities and that the second child who died had contained an evil ghost that had to be exorcized so that it would not reincarnate and come back into the family. Another ritual involved hanging the dead body of the infant from a tree. The ghost could not come back because the body had not touched the ground. Much of this ancient fantasy dwindled by 500 A.D.

Cradles were rarely used. Children would cling to their mothers all day long, particularly while the mother was nursing, which lasted three to four years with no fixed feeding schedule. Feeding was on demand.

The father, meanwhile, had no special duties to the wife or the child. The men were gone for almost half a year, living in the fields away from home in the summertime, or away at work. They had little contact with their young children. But when they could, husbands helped by cooking and doing other chores at home when the mother was nursing the child. This male participation typical among the Chinese was highly unusual in other cultures in ancient times. Chinese men did draw the line at washing clothes, as that was considered women's work.

By the time the male child was older, the father's influence increased markedly, though less so for girls. Children were punished, not by hitting, but by threatening the child with the father. When a child was six years of age it usually collected grass to feed the animals. By the time the girls were 12 they had learned the basic adult tasks, and no longer engaged in children's play. The transition from childhood into adult maturity was a very gradual process. Children learned by example. They were encouraged to mimic their parents.

Arrangements for marriage were usually made when children were six or seven years of age. Among the Chinese books of law, the *Jishi* (Good Rock), also provided for the office of matchmaker (*meishi*), who was required to keep a record of all males and females over three months of age and to instruct the people that men should marry by age 30 and women by 20. Each spring for a month, the *meishi* directed local communities to arrange meetings for men or women who were of age but not yet married. Only during this period was elopement permitted. The *meishi* also arranged for widows and widowers to marry. Later in Chinese history the age of marriage was reduced to 20 for males and 15 for females.

Marriage gifts were given to the girl's family, who returned them to the boy as the girl's dowry. A girl's parents would add to the dowry, depending on their status and wealth.

In early ancient times a son would sometimes be provided with a wife who had been raised with him. Arrangements were sometimes made where an infant girl was adopted into the family by a boy's parents. She would be called "little daughter-in-law" (*simpua*). She was raised as a sibling but married to the son at an appropriate age. Theoretically she was treated as a daughter until the time of her marriage, but often she was treated worse. She was expected to do more work and was frequently the recipient of harsh punishment. In the poorest peasant families a daughter marrying into another family would cause a serious economic loss. The girl's family would lessen their loss by making their daughters work as early as age seven while their brothers were still playing. Another device was to exchange one infant girl for another. The family would then raise the infant girl as a bride for one of their sons, a "little-daughter-in-law."

Patrician life was different. If children were not needed in the fields, the boys were educated and the girls, at age 10, were separated and restricted to the woman's quarters, where they would learn women's duties—obedience, working with hemp, and weaving. When her father arranged her marriage and she became engaged, the girl went to the ancestral temple for three months and was given a new name.

Non-noble girls were given responsibilities sooner than boys. Usually, by the age 5 or 7 girls were responsible for care of a younger child. Boys had no responsibilities until they were sent into an apprenticeship or into the field a year or two later.

No part of the adult world except sexual activity was closed to the growing child. Furthermore, no part of the child's world was exclusively for children. They had no privacy. The richer the parent, the more indulgence the child was shown, for this was the parents' way of proving their affluence and success. Children of the poor learned to be frugal and industrious, while those of the very wealthy often became extravagant and corrupt.[84]

Children entered the adult world much sooner than in other societies. Immaturity and play were not appreciated. Adult behavior was praised. As a result, children developed patterns of behavior such as fear of authority figures, silence, withdrawal, negativism, passive resistance, dampening of emotional expression and activity, and a tendency to assume guilt. Thus, a depressed mode was (and still is) a common symptom among the Chinese. Children were trained to deny their own sense of individuality. At home children were taught to be passive, particularly toward their parents. Hostility was forbidden, no matter what the provocation.

By the 9th century B.C. education existed in district schools where boys lived for nine years (if they were not needed to work in the fields). If the family could afford to keep him there, a boy might extend his education to his tenth or twelfth year. In school he was taught the "rites" and the six sciences (dancing, music, archery, chariot driving, writing, and arithmetic).

After they entered school, children could expect rigorous discipline, usually meted out by the father, who was more likely to discipline his sons than his daughters. They were expected to meet their school responsibilities, and if they did not, they were punished.

Until a child was 10, it was the mother who usually determined the punishment of an errant child. After that, the father disciplined the sons and the mother continued disciplining the daughters. Older brothers could also discipline younger brothers, and in the absence of their mother, occasionally their younger sisters. Rejection was a typical punishment, as was verbal disapproval. Occasionally an errant child would be hit, though severe beating was a rarity and usually the sign of a disturbed father/son relationship.

The worst form of punishment was disinheritance, employed when the child was considered hopeless. One of the most important ways of pressuring youngsters to conform was by confronting them with their genealogical roots. The praiseworthy records of ancestral achievements would be impressed upon them.

But poverty and famine sometimes took their toll on ancient Chinese families and especially on their children. Neither basic education nor formal education in preparation for employment were options always open to the poor.

The poorest families during times of stress and starvation had little choice but to sell their daughters as kitchen slaves, or second wives, to the wealthy; and there was always the last resort of infanticide.

A village was set on an area of cultivated land of approximately 3,065 *mow* (461 acres). If there were 360 households in a typical village, each could only occupy a 9.5 *mow* (1.2 acres) plot for cultivation. Each *mow* would produce about six bushels of rice, and it took 27 bushels of rice to feed one man, woman, and child for one year. Thus, a family group of three needed a piece of land of about 5 *mow*.

As the population exploded in China it became necessary to limit the number of children. A family with only 9 *mow* was in jeopardy of starvation if additional children were born. When the children grew up, before the father died, and particularly afterwards, the property would be divided (fewer *mow*). That resulted in certain poverty and starvation for sons and their families.

The usual solution to this problem was either infanticide or abortion—and infanticide, as we have learned, was generally forbidden. But impoverished Chinese killed unwanted babies. The alternative seemed worse than the crime. It is also true that there was more infanticide of females than males, since the girl was of "less value." The Chinese generally disliked infanticide and abortion and they worked to equalize the land distribution.

A child's life was not always this well ordered. For example, if a child's mother died, the father would often remarry. If he didn't, his children were left with a caretaker whose concern was principally for her own children. Even a stepmother was more interested that her biological children be part of the family lineage. As a result, motherless children were usually the object of discrimination.

In a report given to me (1987) by Lloyd deMause, who has written and researched extensively the issue of child abuse, he stated that in 801 A.D. the West had a male to female ratio of 1.56; in 1391 it was 1.72, in 1750 it was 1.05. In China, in 382 A.D. the male to female ratio was 1.61, in 1760 it was 1.28. According to these figures it would indicate that there was a similar infanticide rate in the East as in the West, though other material seems to challenge this. I believe it is important to remember that females were not always counted in the census, many infants died during childbirth, and more died due to induced abortion and the secondary infections and complications that followed.

This, however, does not deny that females were more depreciated than males in the Chinese culture, and that there was female infanticide.[85,86] Particularly since the 15th century there has been a higher rate of starvation for large segments of the population, so that female infanticide would be much more likely. Wealthy families took more care with all their children and were less likely to practice infanticide.

Going back to early ancient history, from 2500 to 2200 B.C. and even as late as 1000 B.C., there is scant evidence of infanticide. Much did occur because of the belief that certain births were unlucky and that the child had to die. In the most extreme cases, these "unlucky" children were killed. This type of infanticide usually was practiced through exposure. The Chinese literature that describes these cases uses them as examples of what should not be done, warning that a fine person might have lived, had an infant not been killed by its parent.

All Chinese historians note that infanticide did occur, but in early Chinese culture it was invariably related to poverty, famine, or superstition, and was not an established custom. The classic odes referring to families and children never made any reference to infanticide, as in "for ordering of your homes, for joy of child and wife, consider well the truth I tell: this is the charm of life."

During the terrible drought of 801 B.C. or during the 6th century B.C., when China was hit by floods, locusts, and famine, there is no record of children being killed (indicating the number of infanticides were few). But there is a record of infanticide during a siege in 592 B.C. Every example of infanticide and child exposure in classic Chinese literature was written to demonstrate that parents had the power of life and death over their children, and that they should be respected, but that it was not a custom to be followed.

Because of the Chinese reverence for ancestors and the continuation of the line by the next generation, less infanticide existed in this society than in the West.

During the pre-Tang and Tang dynasties, Buddhism flourished in China and many charitable and social welfare activities developed for orphans. In later, traditional China, the literati and gentry took over responsibility for much of this charity work and ran these organizations (free schools, orphanages).

One of the things they attempted to do was to eliminate infanticide, which did not become a major problem in Chinese culture until the 17th century.

Chinese society began to change significantly following the conquest by Genghis Khan.[86] In 1381, in a study of 73,000 households in China the sex ratio in Yun-chou was 126 males to 100 females. In 1572 there were 460 males to 100 females, which indicates an increase in the practice of female infanticide. Though these figures may be somewhat skewed, the general impression of travelers in China in the 1700s and 1800s was that the male population far outnumbered the female—especially in the south. Conditions had so deteriorated in China that by the 17th century it was not only the poor who killed their female infants, but also the wealthy, who feared having to provide large dowries.

It has always been difficult to get an accurate picture of female infanticide in China.[87] The inaccuracy of records was somewhat related to the fact that children were taxed and families sometimes hid or killed their children in order to avoid payment. They killed infants by drowning them in "baby ponds," with immersion in cold or boiling water. At times they would suffocate, strangle, or even bury the infants alive.

From the Former Han to the Later Han Period there was a decided advancement in the culture in terms of its attitude toward infanticide. However, the custom continued sporadically and was noted in the Yan clan of 420 to 489 A.D.

The poet Su Shi (1037-1137 A.D.) joined peers in an effort to stop infanticide. He established a "save the child" association which gave food, clothing, and money to needy expectant mothers, as long as they promised to raise their children. This practice increased during the Mongol dynasty, as did infanticide. There were attempts to establish foundling homes, and Marco Polo noted[88] that 20,000 babies were so raised. The Chinese were oppressed by the Mongols and there was decreased family stability and more infanticide.

The Mongols (Yuan) passed a law aimed at stopping the Chinese from killing their children by ruling that anyone who killed a baby girl was liable to have half his family property confiscated by the army. However, the process continued sporadically even through the Ming period.[89] The famous Italian Jesuit Matteo Ricci noticed in 1610 incidents of female infanticide by drowning. He believed this was due primarily to the fear that a child born into poverty would eventually be enslaved or sold as a concubine. Families desperate for money or food would do such things. The practice increased so that by the 19th century, one governor of Guang Dong province stated that he found the practice of drowning female children common, even among the wealthy. There was significant deterioration of the Chinese attitudes about infanticide starting from the time of the Mongol conquest.

During the Yuan dynasty (Mongol), poorer families had fewer children. One author noted that a man "should have numerous sons but he brings up no more than four and keeps no more than three daughters. At the moment of birth, a bucket of water should be kept ready for drowning the infant immediately. This is called bathing the infant. This practice is commonest at a time in the central regions northwest of Fuchu. Elsewhere this custom is known as harrowing the progeny. Any child born after the inheritance has been divided among the sons was to be drowned."

Clearly, the clan of early ancient China believed that human life was sacred. Murder was an unforgivable crime. People were required to call for help when they saw the life of another in danger. They could not morally or legally justify killing their own infant. All the clan rules were against infanticide, indicating a constant struggle against it. Any poor family that practiced infanticide because of its impoverishment was placed outside the clan and would therefore be under even greater stress than before. But since the clan did not necessarily provide for economic security, if a man were severely impoverished, he might commit infanticide and lose nothing but his social status.

If a father killed a grown son he would be beaten and imprisoned for a year. Though in contemporary times that punishment may seem mild, it was severe for its day and certainly more so than in ancient Greece and Rome. Originally a father in ancient China could sell his family into slavery. This changed by 600 B.C. In fact, the laws regarding treatment of children became more stringent as the Chinese culture matured.

During the 6th century B.C., a minister of state complained that the law prevented him from putting to death a son who had been slanderous to him. In the Han dynasty of 202 B.C. a father could be executed for killing his son, "because human beings are more important than the nature of heaven and earth." Further, the right to kill somebody was the right of an emperor, because the emperor directly or indirectly provided education for the children and therefore was the second father. During the Han dynasty it was illegal to commit infanticide. If a parent killed a child or grandchild in anger with a knife in the 4th century A.D., he would receive five years' imprisonment and punishment. If he beat the child to death he was imprisoned for four years. By the Tang dynasty (618 A.D.), the killing of a son or grandson for any reason was punished by imprisonment. However, it should be noted that a loose-living daughter who was bringing shame upon her clan or ancestors might be killed without punishment to the parent.

As late as the Manchu period,[90] we find many more adult males than adult females. This is not due only to female infanticide, but the more vulnerable girls' response to ordinary childhood illnesses. Female children were made to work at an early age. There was a relatively high rate of female suicide after marriage. Some died in childbirth, but generally because of the enormous workload put on females; they—especially the poor—could be considered the most disadvantaged minority since the Yuan period.

Equally, if not more disadvantaged were the mentally ill.[91-97] Yet the Chinese had a humane attitude to that segment of their society centuries in advance of the West.

Community support of humane attitudes can be seen in the type of medical care provided. There were hospitals for the insane in the capitol by 700 B.C. Furthermore, the reverence for family members, particularly the elderly, led to a general reluctance to institutionalize older persons.

In contrast to some of the more rigorous treatment of the mentally ill in the West, such as dousing and restraints, patients who were brought to a physician for treatment of a mental disorder in ancient China received very different care. Some traditional regimens used were acupuncture, moxibustion, herbal medicines, special forms of massage, and exercises. There were also music and story telling therapies.

The Chinese understanding of psychological problems was sophisticated for this ancient period. They believed that excessive worry and apprehension could injure the heart, which in turn could make the mind weak. People were advised to live up to the principle of Yin/Yang, that is, to be orderly and harmonious in all areas of eating, living, and sex, so as to maintain proper vitality and insure a long life.

In the pre-Chin period (220 B.C.) the treatment for any excited form of insanity—anxiety, manic disorders—was based on the belief that there was an explosion of excessive positive force, which people were encouraged to release. For the Chinese it has always been a virtue to avoid angry expressions. To break such a cultural tradition evoked great shame and disapproval from the family and clan.

China's psychiatric concepts were not influenced by religious thought or religious movements throughout its entire history. Medicine was always separated from sorcery and was seldom influenced by it. The major responsibility for the care of the mentally ill always resided within the family.

(An interesting note about current Chinese Americans is that research has shown that they tend to express psychological conflicts through bodily symptoms more than the general population. They tend to conform more, are less socially extroverted, are more concrete in their approaches to life, and have more depression. This indicates that even though Chinese culture has advanced through many centuries and has been transported into the international mainstream, the ancient Chinese traditions still permeate their homelives.)

In reviewing the Chinese culture one can isolate certain themes. Outstanding is a sense that family is central to one's life. Harmony, moderation, and the avoidance of hostility are other significant characteristics.

The ancient Chinese are perhaps not given enough credit for the astounding contributions they have made to world civilization. They were the inventors, scientists, scholars, and philosophers who shaped much of the world, though the credit for these contributions is often given to Westerners, who have always been more vocal in their quest for fame and fortune.

The Chinese historically have exhibited moderation in all things; excess is non-Chinese. Family organization and respect and care for its members, especially the elderly, is another important characteristic. Literacy, education, and nonviolence have made them a less aggressive and more intellectually oriented people. Their nonrigid (loose) religious attitudes along with their more positive response to women (as central to the family) has been expressed with less child abuse (including infanticide), and a more humane treatment of women and children.

The Chinese, rather, wanted very strongly to survive, culturally and physically. This they did with a remarkable grace and humanity to which the rest of the blossoming world was unaccustomed.

We will explore these and other qualities in a later chapter relative to other societies, particularly as these subjects apply to the treatment of children and women.

Chapter 7

A Comparison of the Five Cultures

*If we cannot see things clearly, let us at least look squarely at
the obscurities.*
Sigmund Freud

Our whirlwind tour of the ancient world has ended and the time
has come for reflection. We have traveled the great Nile through
ancient Egypt. We have walked 40 years with the tribes called
Hebrews to the land known as Israel, and continued on to
Greece and across the Adriatic to Rome. Finally we have visited
China, exploring its development from prehistoric times, and
through the dynasties that introduced great scientific and social
advancements to the rest of the civilized world.

In our travels we have seen glimpses of family life from 4000
B.C. to our own century A.D. This is an inspiring distance to
travel in terms of time and social development. We must absorb
and process a great deal of information if we seek to learn from
the civilizations that preceded our own. The essence of those
distant lands and times is an integral part of our world today.
It is impossible to deny our link with them. Our past is our
present.

In reviewing these five cultures of our ancient past—the

worlds of the Egyptian, Greek, Hebrew, Roman, and Chinese—we find very little information available about the daily family life and childhood of the Egyptian culture. Why is this so?

The ancient Egyptian focused primarily on death and the "life hereafter." Egyptian religion was devoted to an animal anthropomorphic mythology related to death, not life. Therefore, we find that little was written (and little remains) to tell us about their family life and childhood. What little information we do have about families concerns their preparations for their own deaths and rituals for their dead ancestors. Little information exists prior to the Ptolemies about children and family relationships. We can assume that what little information did exist was lost in the destruction of the great library of Alexandria. We are left with papyri of medical and other adult activities, along with hieroglyphics on tomb and temple walls, which make little reference to families and children.

By comparison, there is much more material available about family life and the treatment of children in ancient Greece. However, because children and women were considered relatively unimportant compared with Greek "heroes," a significant discrepancy exists between what was written about women and (especially) children, and the detailed texts describing the "heroic" struggles of men.

We find a similar attitude in Rome: a fixation on war, the profits of conquest, protection of the empire, and the administration of government. Though the Romans showed more interest than the Greeks in their women, little was written about the children of that culture.

Moreover, we should bear in mind that although all three of these societies had chroniclers and historians, they were often more interested in appealing to the authorities and crowds, or furthering their own biases rather then recording the truth. Thus, the accuracy of historical reports about life during ancient times must be questioned. One example is the Greek glorified versions (distortions) of the Persian invasion of Attica, at the battle of Marathon.

We are much better able to study family life and the treatment of children in the two remaining ancient cultures, the Hebrews and the Chinese. These civilizations not only wrote extensively about every aspect of their nation's development, they also placed great emphasis on the family, which was a central theme in both of these cultures. In these societies historians took pride in the accuracy of their accounts. They were noted for their attempt to avoid bias. Although the Chinese often viewed themselves euphemistically and allegorically, so as not to offend the delicate sensibilities within their culture, they recorded their history with all its blemishes visible. The same is true of the Hebrews, who went one step further. The Hebrews used their mistakes as lessons for later generations. They hoped that the world would benefit from their past errors.

Now it is our turn to learn. We must ask ourselves how we will apply the knowledge we have gained of these five cultures to our current understanding of child abuse and the treatment of women in the modern world. Further, with the more advanced knowledge we have today in the areas of psychological and social development we can better understand the motivation and life-styles of these five cultures.

Current knowledge, gleaned from numerous studies of child abuse—studies that we will detail later—tell us that there are certain societal, familial, and personal characteristics that are frequently found in cases of child abuse.

We are apt to find child abuse in a *society*(A) when it exhibits:

1. Aggressive and hostile behavior toward other societies.
2. Loose structure with little respect for individual rights.
3. Low level of responsibility toward those who are needy, sick, or underprivileged.

4. Strong tendency toward transiency.
5. Great disparity between the "haves" and "have nots."
6. Glorification of war.
7. Tolerance for violence and violent games as an important part of childhood play.
8. Acceptance and encouragement of corporal punishment of children.
9. Overcrowding.
10. Group hatred of other groups within or outside of the general society.
11. Rigid and authoritarian religion.
12. Belief in strong or even sadistic punishment of those who violate laws.
13. Extensive pornography.
14. Mythology and literature that portrays women as castrators.
15. Weak sanctions against child abuse.
16. Attitude or social code that supports sexual abuse of women and children.
17. Patriarchal despotism.
18. Lack of emotional, social, and family support for mothers.
19. Marked female inequality in society and family.
20. Disregard for the legal or social rights of children.

We are apt to find child abuse in a *family* (B) when it exhibits:

1. Tendencies to be disrupted and unstable, as in serious verbal and physical fighting, separations, impulsive acting out, and poor parental relations.
2. Economic deprivation.
3. Willingness to have children function to gratify parental needs.
4. Emotional incompatibility between marriage partners.
5. Need to teach children to obey authority in exaggerated ways.

6. Pattern of relationships characterized by domination/submission, where the men dominate.
7. Little male involvement with small children.
8. Family code so stringent that society has little ability to intervene or control the family.

Using these traits as criteria, we can see that some of the societies we have studied easily fit the characteristics. Also, as these societies changed by becoming more warlike and aggressive, by using more severe punishments, or depending on more slaves, they also began abusing their children, and denigrating the roles of women in their cultures.

We recall that Egypt, for example, was the least militaristic country in North Africa and the Middle East, protected and family-oriented, until the time of the New Kingdom (1554-1075 B.C.), when it suddenly became an aggressive empire. Egypt was also a society that did not condone infanticide. Egyptians responded with similar warmth toward daughters and sons and, compared with other societies we have studied, treated men and women as near equals. But we also recall that during times of upheaval, many of these social rules were dropped. Almost immediately infanticide increased and family life deteriorated.

The culture of the Hebrews, on the other hand, was an aggressive and violent culture in its earliest history, biblical and prebiblical, and developed into a peace-seeking nation. Corresponding to their changing attitudes was a new code of morality, a strict one, where family life solidified, infanticide and barbarism ceased, and women became an integral part of Hebrew life.

For centuries the Greeks were devoted to war against other civilizations and among themselves. Theirs was a civilization filled with extreme prejudice. The ancient Greeks enslaved people in other lands, and captives of opposing city-states, and trained their children to fight. This was also a culture in which the incidence of infanticide, child abuse, and denigration of women were commonplace.

Similarly, in ancient Rome, societal orientation was geared towards war and aggression. Rome was a culture that used violence and sadism as forms of entertainment. Child abuse, infanticide, and maltreatment of women were not only tolerated, they were encouraged. They exceeded Greece in every form of adult and child abuse.

By comparison, the ancient Chinese developed a culture that was antimilitaristic. Scholars and philosophers were revered. Soldiers were positioned at the lowest level of society. The Chinese society deplored violence, and as a result, rates of infanticide, child abuse, and female denigration were comparatively low.

Using our list as a reference, we can see very clearly that where each of the societal or familial characteristics indicative of child abuse was evident, infanticide and child abuse increased.

Let us then take one more look at the ancients before turning to modern times.

The Egyptians: A civilization whose treatment of children was generally benign, whose family life was strong, and whose view of women, as compared to other civilizations in the area at the time, was relatively fair.

In terms then, of child abuse among the ancients, the Egyptians were not major offenders:

1. Slavery was never a major aspect of Egyptian civilization.
2. Child abuse and infanticide rates were relatively low.
3. The civilization itself was stable, though, as in all civilizations, during times of strife infanticide and child abuse increased.
4. The culture displayed a social awareness through its religion.
5. Early in their history the Egyptians showed interest in

psychology and an awareness of the diseases and ills of mankind and how to cure them.

6. The Egyptians were terrified of their gods, and did not see them as loving.
7. The Egyptians showed extensive interest in death, dying, and mourning: an indication of an ability to love. Loving one's parents in life means a loss at their death. The freedom to feel and express these feelings is seen in a full mourning process (sobbing, etc.). Full mourning tends to prevent melancholia.
8. Monogamous marriages were the rule and family life was stable.
9. They had an extensive educational system for boys, a lesser one for girls.
10. They followed laws that protected both women and children.
11. The Egyptians allowed great sexual freedom, nudity to seminudity of children up to the age of puberty, and freedom to engage sexually until the time of marriage. This demonstrates a less rigid punitive structure and more warmth and equality for women.
12. Mothers had a close relationship with their children and there was little separation or abandonment of children.

The Greeks: A civilization whose values centered on war and violence; a civilization in constant turmoil where infanticide rates were high and women were generally denigrated.

Among the five civilizations we have studied, Greece was among the worst offenders toward women and children:

1. The Greeks had extensive slavery, which was essential to their economy. They devalued a person's worth by enslaving him. Slavery increased in this society until the end of their civilization.
2. Greece had a glaring history of child abuse (sexual and nonsexual), violence toward children, and infanticide.

No society except Rome equaled or exceeded it for its cruelty and abuse of children.

3. They showed less disparity between the "haves" and "have nots" in their earliest history. Later, the disparity grew to such an extent that the society was in danger of revolution and disruption.
4. They often killed the mentally ill or disadvantaged by sacrificing them to the gods.
5. Greek gods were harsh, destructive, and vindictive. They arbitrarily lied and cheated and demanded sacrifices.
6. The Greeks celebrated the death of heroes, though sometimes were so angry with the loss that instead of lamenting they would become enraged and slaughter the enemy as a sacrifice to the dead loved one.
7. They began civilization with a concept of love in marriage, but as the civilization matured, marriage was considered only for the purpose of creating heirs. Women were severely denigrated.
8. Education was a privilege of the few; but for a few exceptions, females were excluded.
9. The Greeks had few laws that protected women and children and no consistently stable legal system. Infanticide and sacrifice were not condemned by law.
10. They began civilization with sexual freedom; however, later they isolated and sexually restricted women. Men had extensive sexual freedom to abuse children, practice homosexuality, perform castration, and employ boy prostitutes.
11. Women were severely depreciated and suppressed. As a result they devoted little attention to the care of their children and passed most of the responsibility on to the slaves.

The Hebrews: A civilization whose values were built upon a strong moral code which protected the rights of women and children and supported family unity.

Of the five civilizations we have studied, the Hebrews treated women and children the best:

1. The bonded person was not considered a nonperson and had extensive rights, including the right to obtain freedom.
2. Though there was infrequent and episodic infanticide, this was always abjured and not part of society's mode of functioning. Generally their culture was the most benign in the care of children.
3. A homogeneous group of people throughout their history, the Hebrews maintained a continuous stable society.
4. The Hebrews showed extensive understanding of the psychological problems of the mentally ill and did not punish them for their illness or problems.
5. They were a God-intoxicated people, whose God went from being a powerful and avenging Jehovah to a more benign, loving, protective God in the transition from the early biblical to the Talmudic period. Human sacrifice and violence was considered a sin against God.
6. They practiced complicated mourning that involved sadness, crying, and societally supported expressions of unhappiness. This allows a working through of the loss of love, the prevention of melancholia, and the eventual ease of remembering the loved ones with joy and warmth.
7. The Hebrews maintained strong central orientation around the family and marriage. Good marriages were a requirement of functioning acceptably in the society.
8. More than any other civilization, the Hebrews stressed education for girls and boys.
9. They established an extensive legal system that was intimately a part of the religious system.
10. They allowed extensive sexual freedom prior to marriage by the male and, to some degree, the female,

though if she was not a virgin she would have difficulty getting an appropriate husband. Sexual activity was not only permitted but encouraged, and women had a greater right to sexual fulfillment than men.

11. They fostered a positive attitude about women in later history, but earlier were deprecatory toward them. The Hebrews considered the care of the mother and child vital and central to their culture.

The Romans: A civilization which was warlike, violent, depreciative of women and children, and practiced infanticide and child abuse to excess.

Of the five civilizations we studied, Rome competed with Greece as one of the worst offenders in child abuse and negative attitudes toward women:

1. Slavery was extensive and cruel. The Romans employed armies to control their slave populations.
2. The Romans extensively abused children, though the proportion of infanticide and sexual abuse never quite reached that found in Greece.
3. Despite its huge empire, Rome had little social awareness. An increasing disparity existed between the "haves" and "have nots." No attempt was made to improve the lot of the poor or unfortunate.
4. They mistreated and sacrificed the mentally ill and poor.
5. Roman gods were cruel and demanded human sacrifices. The Romans, who were extremely superstitious, embraced the gods of the lands they conquered.
6. The Romans responded to the death of a hero with pomp and circumstance, as well as the sacrifice of enemy victims.
7. In early Rome marriages were unions of affection, but by the late empire this had deteriorated greatly, until married and family life was severely denigrated.
8. Education was primarily for boys and for the purpose of

administration, war, and conquest. Wealthy Romans sent their children to Greece to be educated.

9. The legal system gave no protection to children and very little to women.
10. Extensive sexual activity was allowed, and carried into pornography, sadism, and debauchery.
11. Although women were given more freedom in Rome than in Greece, motherhood was depreciated and there was less care for children, with more instances of abandonment and abuse.

The Chinese: This vast civilization honored scholars and despised war. Family life was central to the development of the culture and women were treated as near-equal to men.

Of the five civilizations we have studied, China is among the best in its treatment of children and women:

1. China had a history of slavery, but it was not as extensive as other cultures and slave abuse did not usually occur. It did arbitrarily enslave criminals and their entire families. Captives taken in war were enslaved as well.
2. The Chinese history of infanticide virtually ceased by 200 B.C., when human sacrifice also was eliminated. Infanticide began to increase again in the 17th century A.D.
3. The Chinese nation has been the most homogeneous, stable, intact culture in the history of the world.
4. There was a large middle class comprised of educated people of modest means.
5. The Chinese sometimes hid or killed the mentally ill so that their defect would not reflect badly upon the family. However, the mentally ill and the unfortunates were generally well-protected. The more secure the family (clan) the more likely they would protect the emotionally ill.
6. As the civilization developed, the Chinese became less

and less religiously oriented. Instead, they developed a "religion" built on moral concepts. There was an extensive belief in an afterlife but not in direct relationship to any particular god. It was a philosophical position more than a religion.

7. They practiced extensive mourning rituals which included signs of sincere sadness. Since depression was such an accepted attitude in China, melancholia was a much more common social experience. The Chinese felt it wise to hide their emotions.

8. Marriage was always of central importance in maintaining family continuity. Marriages were stable and affection between husband and wife was the rule.

9. The Chinese were devoted to education for boys and girls.

10. By 200 B.C. there was a well-established codification of the law which gave extensive protection to women and children.

11. China allowed great sexual freedom within the marital relationship. Men had much sexual freedom outside the home as a result of organized prostitution. Women had more rights and freedom to participate sexually with other women and their husbands than men.

12. China always made the mother's role central and gave her special deference because of the responsibility she had for the heir of the family. Though the status of woman was inferior to man's, it was not without importance. In the home, woman was central. Outside the home, she was inferior and unimportant.

Thus concludes our overview of civilizations past. But what conclusions can we draw from the study of ancient cultures?

It is apparent that neither the level of scientific or industrial development nor the amount of wealth have determined which societies will abuse their children. Egypt's wealth, Grecian civilization, and Roman power did not prevent child abuse. The poverty and powerlessness of the Diaspora Jews did not produce child abuse. The power and wealth of Renaissance Europe did not prevent child abuse. China, despite despots, tyrants, and barbarian incursion and conquest, maintained a family cohesion and less child abuse until the 17th century.

In our next chapter we will utilize our scientific knowledge and understanding to explore our world, the family, and child care in the modern world. In the last chapter, applying the lessons of the past and that knowledge, we will approach today's most dangerous threat to the heart of America's family unit.

Chapter 8

The Psychodynamics of Child Abuse

> *The child is father of the man.*
> Wordsworth

Why do we find child abuse incomprehensible in the modern age? Why do we believe it is a local or temporary aberration? Historical evidence shows us that child abuse is neither a local problem, nor a temporary state of affairs.

In our sophisticated modern world, sociologists, psychiatrists, psychologists, psychoanalysts, and child specialists have studied and reached general agreement about the characteristics and dynamics of violence, family abuse, and child abuse.

By analyzing the traits of individuals who are prone to commit child abuse, we can see that in our own modern society it is not difficult to recognize how we continue, in some quarters, to follow philosophies and codes that make child abuse a natural extension of our attitudes and actions. Up to this point we have examined and compared in great detail the ancient cultures and how they treated their children. Certain features of the ancient societies prevailed in those most abusive to children. Still, within any given society there are those more predisposed to violence than others. Let us now look at those traits in individuals that predispose them more to child abuse. We will examine these traits within the context of our own modern society. (In the concluding chapter we will compare the ancients' cultures with our modern society to draw some conclusions on how modern America's mores and norms fit into the pattern of perpetuating child abuse through the ages.)

In modern times, we often read about children being murdered, tortured, and neglected. What drives an individual to perpetrate such heinous acts?

An individual is apt to commit child abuse when he or she:[A]

1. has weakened behavioral controls, for example, as a result of the episodic use of drugs or alcohol which can impair judgment;
2. is a lying parent;
3. is sadistic to the child and to outsiders;
4. shows hostility toward children within the home and outside it, generally including victimization;
5. has poor self-esteem (particularly the mother);
6. lacked affection or had an erratic upbringing in early childhood;
7. is undereducated;
8. has few employable skills;
9. as a mother, directs her sons to act like little men;
10. is depressed and feels hopeless about the future;
11. is less nurturing;
12. is impulsive;
13. is socialized to see sexual activity as separate from the marital or loving relationship;
14. is taught that a sex object is smaller, weaker, and inferior;
15. as a parent, is punitive to daughters about sexual matters;
16. thinks the sexual act is a way to dominate another person;

17. is a parent who is absent from child care;
18. is ambivalent toward children;
19. sees the world irrationally as a dangerous place; and/or
20. is a man who functions better in relationships with other mens' sons than with his own.

(Women more than men abuse children under the age of three. Men more than women abuse children over the age of three, the latter being true of child abuse by much older children.)

Among all mammals,[1] the only exception being humans, infants tend to be killed by unrelated individuals. Only in the human species is the mother the killer of her own infant. In primate societies the infanticidal male is never the father of any infant he kills, and the killer males invariably kill to gain sexual access to the mother sooner than if the infant had lived.

Among mice, a male familiar with the mother is not likely to kill her offspring, even if he is not the father. In the study of most mammals, fathers cause more harm to their offspring when they have not been paired with the mother in a monogamous arrangement (except for primates). There is no case among wild monkeys where a mother has killed her own offspring. Murderous abuse by mothers is only found in captive primates, particularly among those who have been most socially isolated. Studies of humans show contrary evidence. There is greater danger from intimate members of the family, particularly from mothers of children under one year of age.

Much, but not all child abuse has a violent quality. Besides actual physical abuse (which includes infanticide) we find abandonment, rejection, sexual abuse, restrictions (restraints, swaddling, food deprivation, limitation of freedom), oppression (depreciations, forced ignorance), and slavery (including premature and/or oppressive work situations). Understanding these behaviors is most difficult. However, we will look at some of the sociopsychological factors that make up the violent individual as well as more specific areas of child abuse.

To prepare for this, let us first look at what normal child

development should be like.[2-4] Clinicians and researchers since at least the time of Sigmund Freud and other investigators of human development have shown that the first five years are crucial in human development. They have emphasized the prime and vital significance of the mother in the development of the child, particularly prior to age three. The literature and research to support this belief is extensive.

Studies have repeatedly shown that though fathers do have a certain significance in a child's development under three years, the prime figure is the mother. Even when fathers are significant and available during this period, it is always the mother who is viewed as the primary giver and protector by the child.

Reports of childhood depression, autism, and schizophrenia clearly demonstrate the importance of a mother's psychic state in relation to the very young child. The studies of anorexia nervosa/bulimia also indicate the significance of mother's emotional state as well as the way she responds to the very young female child as being determinants for this illness.

The most important aspect of a child's development in the first six to twelve months of life is the need for a mother who is there almost constantly and instantly providing warmth, affection, succor, and aid. The physical care of the child is not enough. The child clearly needs the warm, happy, comfortable, and calm response of the mother.

After the first few weeks of life the child can respond to the quality of mothering it receives and can sense the tension of the maternal figure. There is something about the type of personality, internal comfort, and security of the mother that makes it possible for her to provide the happiest stable environment possible for her child.

Another fact that has been established by animal and human studies is that from infancy on, and certainly by the age of two, a child's personality and behavior has been formed, based more on the imitation of its mother's actions than those of any other figure. That is true for boys and for girls. Thus, who mother is and how she responds to the child, as well as how she responds to herself, will determine how the child, in a mirrorlike fashion, will establish its own identity.

By the third year of life, a child is so well socialized that he has learned not only his sex and gender, but understands relationships between genders to a significant degree. He has adequate language skills. He also has an accurate idea of his position in relation to the family unit and to the extended family unit, as well as to some of the peripheral social contacts in his environment around the home. He may have begun to establish even more extended social contacts in nursery school or larger group play activities.

Between ages three and five, all the complexities of the oedipal (family) relationship come into play. In a complex social way this demonstrates mother and father's relationship to each other and defines the roles and relationships between men and women. The oedipal complex deals with passive, aggressive, and sexual feelings. Assuming the situation has been normal up to three years of age, the child may still have difficulties during this period that can have permanent effects requiring therapeutic measures.

It is obvious that during this period the relationship between mother and father is crucial in establishing for the child a notion of who he is and how he should respond socially in the complex world. It is at this time that the child learns how to behave with women. The resolution of the oedipal period in the homosexual period of identification that occurs between five and seven years solidifies and puts into practice what the child learned earlier when he or she identifies with the parent of the same sex. Girls identify with mothers and their role and boys identify with fathers and their role. This is achieved by the close loving relationship between the same-sex parent and child.

There is a secondary oedipal period, during the pre- and pubertal period (12 to 14 years of age). It is clear by our more current studies that the latency period (7 to 12 years of age) is a period where the child utilizes group identifications with the same sex as a means of establishing personal identity and relationships to the opposite sex.

If we understand clearly the absolute, final, and central significance of mother's role in a child's development, we will be better equipped to understand child abuse in the past and, more importantly, in our present world.

It is well known by those who work in agriculture, animal and vegetable, that the way a crop is cultivated will determine the quality of produce. Proper nurture of the young seed, young plant, or young animal, is vital in order to achieve a successful outcome. Thus, the farmer or herder takes great care of his vital product. Historically this lesson seems to have been lost in terms of how we care for our children.

The final result of all the evidence is clear to me, not only as an analyst, but also as an historian. It is my view and the conclusion of my research that our whole world revolves around the newborn female, clearly the most important person in the world. I will discuss this further in the final chapter. Those societies that depreciate women to any degree are going to have an increased frequency of child abuse as well as the pathology that results. A society that in any way creates an image of the female child and subsequently the female adult as depreciated, inferior, and inadequate, is going to increase significantly the pathology of child abuse.

If a woman filled with hurt, rage, and self-depreciation has a female child with whom she identifies, she is going to pass along these same negative feelings to her offspring. She will have an untold amount of rage toward her male child, since unconsciously in her mind he represents the male world that has caused all her suffering. It is extremely difficult for a mother who is filled with self-hatred, depression, damaged self-esteem, or borderline psychotic ego construction (as a result of abuse in her own developing years) to be the warm, giving, and nonabusive mother she needs to be for her child.

We have reviewed a history of child abuse and parental behavior as seen in five ancient civilizations. If we were to find one central idea to be drawn from this material, it would be this. How the female is treated and viewed in a particular culture determines the future of that society. A society that appreciates the value of women and realizes their central importance in developing the entire community, beginning with the family unit, will be a society that has the ability to direct its attentions to all matters in a humane, kind way.

Let us look at some facts from our own society:[B]

Currently, in America, 20% of the population approve of a husband and wife hitting each other and, not surprisingly, child abuse is 72% higher in families where the parents approve of slapping their spouses. Accordingly, 30% of child abuse takes place in families where there was an incident of physical violence between parents during the preceding year. When social approval of violence within a family increases, these destructive qualities are transferred to child rearing.

Studies show that the battered woman is more likely to abuse her own child. These women undergo a cycle of violence that has three basic phases:

1. Tension building, during which there are minor physical and verbal assaults upon her. The woman does not protest too strongly, letting the batterer, her husband, know that she will accept his behavior. Tension increases and violence escalates.
2. Battering, where both partners realize they are without control and a severe beating ensues. This may be provoked to get over the tension seen in phase 1.
3. Reconciliation, where the batterer is contrite and the battered woman accepts his pleas for forgiveness. At this point she is a complete victim in that she knows what is going to happen next, but denies it.

Observations have been made of increased violence toward women during pregnancy with the abdomen being the prime target and face and breasts as secondary targets of assault. Studies show that 45% of battered women come from families where the mother was subtly controlling and the father acted as a figurehead authority. Also, 28% of battered women came from families with emotionally disturbed mothers who had many mates, all of whom tended to be somehow abusive. The daughters in these families who later become mothers themselves are looking for a fantasy father whom they don't find. They have developed a "learned helplessness."

In families where a child is abused[5,6] the parents often respond to the child in an unexpected manner. It is as if they are trying to get the child to gratify their own dependent needs—a role reversal. These parents have poor self-esteem and disturbed identifications. Any injury to this fragile self-esteem immediately requires a compensatory adaptation, and they tend to project their problems onto the child. It is as if the child within the parent is the one who is crying and needs to be silenced.

In looking at the sociohistorical characteristics[7] of violent individuals,[8] violent families are most likely to act out (62%) during the premenstrual period. When they were children, these same violent individuals experienced sensory deprivation, lack of affection, erratic childhood supervision, brutality and physical punishment, promiscuity without affection, and humiliation. Violent individuals tend to feel helpless and passive in what they perceive as an oppressive life situation. Their identity is confused. Usually, prior to the violence there is a sudden loss of self-esteem, a sense of being put down. The abuser is usually undereducated with few skills to improve his or her feelings of self-worth.

Socially, the violent individual comes from a society where he is told to hit first before being hit, where war is glorified, and violence in games and toys is an important part of childhood development as presented by parents. Mothers tend to direct their sons to act "like little men."

In our studies we find that conscience[9-12] first comes into play at about one year of age. This early conscience deals with the concept of a primitive *no*. The danger of breaking a rule for the early conscience is an immediate retaliation by the conscience. One way of dealing with the fear of being overwhelmed by one's aggressive impulses and retaliation is to take in and identify with the parent's approach to life; particularly the parent of the same sex. The danger for normal development is continuation of the primitive *no* response past age three or four, producing a rigid punitive conscience. The rigid conscience is normal at two, not later. By identifying with the more realistic and benign attitudes of the parents at age three and beyond there is modification of the earlier more primitive conscience.

The child's early identification with parents, which arises out of an attempt to resolve one's aggressive impulses, develops into a multitude of realistic and distorted images. How you see yourself represented (with distortions) determines how you will respond to the world. In adults, physical aggression that is not a response to a clear threat or unusual provocation is expressed mainly by people with mental illness or severe character disorders. In such instances, the aggression can be attributed either to a pathological intensification of aggressive tendencies (something that is stimulating more aggression) or a weakness of the mind's control mechanism, the ego. Anything that stimulates aggression too much or weakens the control system (the ego) may release destructive behavior; that is, a return to early childhood techniques of responding to the environment.

Parents who lie will produce children who deny.[13] This is one of the fundamental principles of understanding pathology. If a parent lies about reality, children will learn to deny reality. Any distortion of reality presented by parents is perceived by the child as reality in the first few years of life. The world parents create is the young child's only reality. Everything else is unreal. As an adult he will always unconsciously try to recreate the world as he originally perceived it. If the preschool child is not loved or given enough security, he will have an imperfectly developed ego and will likely operate on a primitive conscience level as he grows older. In other words, he will go backward, looking for answers learned during the first years of life.

Children enjoy breaking objects. The child's aggressive, destructive impulses are tied up with hostility. One can derive pleasure from being hostile in a safe setting. However, if the child does not have an appropriate channel for expressing aggression, then it will be directed back against himself. In this case the child's ego must find a way to cope with the self-directed aggression. He or she may manifest this self-aggression as depression, even to the extent of suicide. Another means of dealing with the unexpressed aggression is for the ego to regress to a more primitive level where the aggressive energy is soaked up by moving back, turned against the self. There is an avoidance of reality, a creating of a private world. This is psychosis. Another coping mechanism is murder, in which the individual no longer channels this aggressive behavior at himself, but now, in a disturbed way, protects himself from a projected (imagined) external danger.

Psychosocial Profiles of Violence[14-19]

It was found during a 1953 study[20] of Ceylon that the looser a society structure, and the less respect given to citizen rights and duties, the greater the chance for violence. A. L. Porterfield and R. H. Filbert[21] reported in *Crime, Suicide, and Social Well-Being* that those (U. S.) states with low ratings of social awareness and services (programs for children, aged, infirm, orphans, etc.) have a higher homicide rate. J. P. Humphrey and H. J. Kupferer's[86] study of the southern United States (*Pockets of Violence: An Exploration of Homicide and Suicide*) showed a higher "criminal homicide and assaultive behavior" rate than the rest of the country. They found that those areas of the southeast with high rates of homicide had higher proportions of blacks to whites, less stable populations with more migration, more family disruptions (divorce), more economic deprivation, and more disparity between incomes of blacks and whites. They summarized their findings as follows: "A combination of socio-economic factors which" inhibits social freedom "through economic deprivations and family instability tend to result in more homicidal behavior." When a person is blocked by his society as a result of deprivation or an unstable family background, he is more likely to exhibit homicidal behavior.

If we examine individual cases of violence,[23] certain personal and social facts attract our interest. For example, murder by minors[24,25] seems associated with a transmission of the urge to kill from the parent to child. When the child kills the parent, one of the parents has in some manner urged the child to commit that murder.

The social and historical characteristics of violent[26,27] individuals show some interesting elements: (1) They often have a history of dangerous aggressive driving, with repeated traffic violations and serious accidents. Some may become so terrified of their destructive urges that they are afraid to drive. (2) They may try to act out inappropriate impulses commonly sadomasochistic in type, such as hurting others or themselves, e.g. spouse abuse. (3) Their violence decreases with age. (4) They are usually males between 15 and 24 years old. (5) During their childhood we see behavior that is not age-appropriate including tantrums, explosive behavior, cruelty to young children or animals, antisocial acts, disregard for other's welfare, disruptive behavior in class, inability to function in school, enuresis, and acts of setting fires (after the age of four). (6) Violent females are most likely to act out during their premenstrual period. (7) As children, violent individuals have usually experienced sensory deprivation, lack of affection, erratic childhood supervision, brutality in physical punishment, promiscuity without affection, or humiliation. (8) They tend to feel helpless and passive in what they perceive as an oppressive and hopeless situation. (9)

They fail to develop a clear-cut identity. (10) They tend to be loners, with a lack of success in life for which they blame others. (11) Prior to the violence a loved one commonly threatens to leave or becomes interested in someone else. The individual experiences a sudden loss of self-esteem, a sense of being "put down," and there may be an increase in physical and/or psychological symptoms, such as impotence or depression. (12) They are usually undereducated with few employable skills. (13) They are sullen, negative, and recalcitrant.

If a social situation condones violence, the violence will occur. For example, if hatred felt toward one group is encouraged and accepted by a group, violence against members of the hated group is likely to occur. Where there is overcrowding, no escape is left to release immediate pressure and violence usually follows. Similar situations occur all the time, whether it takes place in a tenement family or a nontenement family on a vacation confined in the small quarters of a tent or cottage. Where there is a subculture of violence within the community or neighborhood (less verbal solutions presented), there tends to be more violence. Where the youth cohorts would rather fight than flee, assault instead of talk, and kill rather than hurt, there will be greater violence.

Thus, if we are to assemble the best predictors of severe violence, they would be: history of past violence, threats of violence, parental deprivation, enuresis past childhood, fire setting in childhood, cruelty to animals or other children in childhood, abuse of barbiturates or alcohol, threat of loss of self-esteem or of love object, availability of a weapon.[28]

Physical Child Abuse[29]

These violent behaviors are promoted by the society at large. Studies of child beating in the United States show that 70% or more of the victims are under three years of age and 32%

are under six months. Another study shows that 60% are under nine months of age. Thus, the vast majority of children that are abused are under three years of age with a significant clustering under one year.

In all the sociological studies there seems to be a close relationship between poverty and various forms of child abuse and neglect. The vast majority of the cases occur in poverty or near-poverty circumstances. Child neglect (inadequate supervision, feeding, etc.) is a much more pervasive problem than the actual physical abuse. There are at least twice as many cases of child neglect (which is primarily not loving the child) than physical abuse; and child neglect seems to be even more related to poverty than child abuse.

In one recent large representative study,[30] some characteristics were compiled describing families where maltreatment (abuse and neglect) occurred:

1. 43 of the 45 families studied were one-parent families headed by women.
2. 53%, that is 24 of the families, were black; 42%, or 19 families, were white; 4%, 2 families, were Puerto Rican.
3. The average number of children per family was between four and five, with 42% of the families, 19 of the 45, having five or more children.
4. In 53% of the families, the main caretaker had a severe physical illness or condition.
5. 76% of the families had at least one child with a serious physical health problem.
6. In 53% of the families the main caretakers (mothers) had spouses or ex-spouses or paramours who produced serious problems for the family: for example, they physically abused the mothers and children, or perhaps used family funds to buy alcohol or drugs.
7. 29% of the mothers indicated they had been severely beaten themselves as children. In almost all of the cases,

the mother was involved directly in abuse of the child. If the spouse was the perpetrator, the mother was usually indirectly involved; she either encouraged or stood by and watched.

It is interesting to note that 16% of these white families were living in deprived or below-average financial circumstances compared with 50% of the black families. What is important about this finding is that, as noted, 53% of the families were black and 42% were white; this means that the economic situation was much better for the whites, yet they seemed to be much more prone to violence. This further indicates that the black families, although under greater stress, seemed better able to cope with the hardship of economic deprivation than white families. Still, it would be accurate to state that material deprivation seems to be related to child abuse as an additional stress. Of these families, 35% lived in deprived material circumstances. The abuse in these families was very severe (major physical injury), compared to the 14% living in less deprived circumstances.

Another finding that is not surprising shows that material deprivation was greater among larger families, as well as those who lived within the highest population density. Two patterns emerged from the study of families on public assistance who abused their children. In one group, the families who lived in the most deprived material circumstances were large and had less contact with a significant male. They resided in decaying, high-density urban areas, and were mostly black, with parents and children who had a variety of physical problems. The severity of maltreatment in these families was greater and their family condition was less likely to improve. The other pattern portrayed families who lived in less severe material deprivation and had fewer children. Proportionally, there were more white families in this group, living in suburban rural communities as well as in central urban areas. The parents and children were less likely to suffer from physical illness. The degree of physical maltreatment in these families was less severe and their condition was more likely to improve with intervention. The children in these families were more likely to have behavioral problems and the parents were likely to have severe emotional and psychological difficulties. Neglect, as opposed to physical maltreatment, was more likely to occur.

Race of Abused Children

Patricia T. Schlosser, in her study *The Abused Child* (1964),[31] found that the racial background of abused children was no different from the general population, while Betty Simmons and Eleanor Downs in their study *Child Abuse Survey* (1966),[32] found a much higher proportion of nonwhites among the abused children. According to Simmons and Downs, fewer than 22% were white, 27% Puerto Rican, and 48% nonwhite. The Brandeis Press survey looked at the racial background of abused children and showed that of 36 fatally injured children, 26 were white and 10 were nonwhite. Of 30 nonfatally injured children, 15 were white and 15 nonwhite. Clearly, there are no consistent findings related to race.

Religion

In 1965, the National Opinion Research Center (NORC)[33] conducted a survey studying the religious background of child abuse victims. In this study no mother who was Jewish, whether the father was Jewish or not, fatally injured a child. When examining the injured child's family it was discovered that in 27% of the families both parents were Protestant. In 22% of the families both parents were Catholic. Of the mixed families, 15% had Catholic mothers and non-Catholic fathers. In 2% of the cases the mother was Protestant and the father was not. Where the mother was Catholic and the father was Jewish, the figure was also 2%. If religion was not known, but was narrowed down to either Catholic or Protestant, 31% of these families abused their children. Clearly this indicates that there is something in the cultural background in most Jewish families that modifies significantly the tendency toward child abuse.

There is a fascinating side note to our historical review and culture comparisons. I am referring to the interesting statistics about Chinese-Americans and Jewish-Americans (second generation or more). These two unrelated ethnic subgroups have similar findings in the relative (percentage of population) absence of any of the forms of child abuse, spouse abuse, community violence (e.g., robbery, murder, rape, rioting, etc.), and mental hospital commitment, as well as a lower incidence of drug and alcohol abuse. Other ethnic subgroups do not demonstrate these same characteristics.

Family and Education

The families of the abused children in the NORC[34] survey showed that most parents were married or had parental substitutes living in the home. Only 15% were single-parent families. In looking at the educational background of the mothers when they were not the sole head of households—that is, there was a husband or father available to head the unit—if the mother completed four years of grade school, only 2.5% were abusers. If the mother completed between five and eight years of school, 15% were abusers. If they had some high school, 12% were abusers. More than 29% of abusers were high school graduates. If they did not complete college, 2.5% were abusers. But out of all college graduates, none were found to be abusers. We are probably observing the self-esteem of mothers. It is likely that these mothers who completed only four years of grade school dropped out to help their mother at home with younger children. Her self-esteem may have been enhanced by identifying with her mother who probably appreciated her. The school dropout later may well be indicating a different phenomenon, namely the upset/depressed girl-teen. Especially is this likely to be the case if they drop out one year short of high school graduation, or drop out after they make it to college. Generally speaking, college graduates comprise a more emotionally stable group than their sister dropouts.

General Parental Characteristics[35-39]

A superficial examination of characteristics of parents (as noted in the NORC survey and other studies) who abuse their children seems to indicate they are not much different from what we would find in a random selection of a dozen people in society. They cover all socioeconomic strata, from the unemployed to the working class, and upwards to the highest professional. They range from the poorest to the wealthiest, though most are in average circumstances. They lived in all kinds of communities from the largest metropolitan area to some of the smallest rural suburbs, with a variety of different housing. IQs range from borderline 70 to the superior rating of 130 or more. The parents' ages range between 18 and 40.

Upon careful examination of family units, however, some interesting points appear. Since the great majority of abusive parents are in marriages that appear relatively stable, closer examination of these marriages show that it was not truly a love relationship that was happy and cooperative. More often there was a desperate clinging together of two dependent people who feared loneliness and loss. The partners were incompatible, with extensive friction, yet shared a desperate need for each other.

Studies show that abusive mothers were often in great need of support from their husbands. The husbands were found to be needy and dependent themselves—unable clearly to express themselves and at the same time demanding, critical, and un-heeding of the mother's needs. There was poor communication between the abusing parents. Despite the fact that they were aggressive, hostile, and destructive to their own children, they showed little aggression and hostility in their relationships out-side the home.

Of those who were involved in their religion, a higher per-centage were strong, rigid, authoritarian fundamentalists in their adherence to their beliefs. Most were Anglo-Saxon; there were no immigrants in the group and true alcoholism was not a problem, though there was evidence of symptomatic excess drinking.

Another and most important characteristic about child abuse is who does what and at what age. When the child is under one year of age, it is almost invariably the mother who is the abuser. In a study of 57 abused children, in 50 instances the mother was the attacker, as opposed to the seven cases where the father was the abuser.

Response of Parents[40-42]

Studies show that the child abuser often has a history of being significantly depressed, episodically. Though they have significant emotional problems requiring treatment, they are not grossly psychotic in the vast majority of cases. Their general attitude toward life is that it is generally hopeless, and they don't think it worthwhile or possible to seek help. They do not feel that they would get a positive response from their environ-ment or support for the difficulties they are in.

Child abusers typically expect and demand a great deal from their infants and children. This is done prematurely, be-yond the ability of the infant or child. It is as if the child is being treated as an adult, and is required to parent the parent. The parent feels insecure, unsure of being loved, and turns to the child as a source of this reassurance and comfort—a role reversal.[43]

The abused child is often seen as a hated part of the abusive parent that the parent wishes to control or destroy. In some cases parents are immature, and resent the dependent demands of the child. They project most of their problems onto the child, believing that the child is the cause of their troubles. Common expressions of abusive parents are: "If you give in to the kids they'll be spoiled rotten." "You have to teach children to obey authority." "I don't want my kids to grow up to be delinquent." "Children have to be taught respect for their parents." Though these thoughts are expressed by nonabusing, as well as abusing parents, the difference seems to be that the abusing parent exaggerates these standards and applies them to younger children. It is possible to conclude that the abuser of children requires infants and children to satisfy their needs; while the needs of the children are disregarded.

The typical abusive parent[44-50] is a married mother, 25 to 30, who was abused as a child and lives in a constant state of marital strife, socially isolated, with financial problems.

Abusive parents often expand the mythology of our society, blowing it out of proportion: for example, the fantasy of baby as a bundle of joy, the mother as madonna, and the concept "spare the rod and spoil the child." Certainly these ideas contain some element of truth (and are culturally accepted), but the abusive parent takes them to bizarre extremes.

We have concluded from a variety of studies of abusing parents that, without exception, parents rear their children as they were brought up themselves. Though some were not severely beaten, all have usually experienced a sense of intense, continuous, and unreasonable demands from their parents. They were expected to be "good" and submissive, "obedient," free of "mistakes," a comfort to their distressed parents, and approving of their parents' actions and behavior even while they were punished. These demands were not only excessive, they were premature. Along with these demands came the parental criticism that the child was always inadequate, inept, ineffectual, and unlovable. All the parents who abused their children were deprived emotionally of basic nurturing when they were children. They were uncared for from the very beginning of their lives. Not only were the parents somehow abused as children by deficient mothering, but the grandparents were as well. Child abuse is like a plague, transmitted from parent to child, pseudogenetic.

It is interesting to note that a landmark article revealing the battered child syndrome appeared July 7, 1962, and was widely disseminated to the public. Since then, however, the underlying characteristics and problems that lead to the syndrome still have not been dealt with, though the problem is more clearly recognized. Following are some of the basic findings from that article[51] about the battered child and the abusive parents:

> "1. Such parents were usually not parented well themselves, often were themselves victims of abuse, are isolated, do not trust others, and have unrealistic expectations of children.
> 2. A child usually exhibits some behavior which the parent correctly or incorrectly, justifiably or unjustifiably, perceives as aversive, and as requiring some intervention to change.
> 3. There is a stressful situation or incident that serves as a trigger.
> 4. The family lives in a culture in which corporal punishment is sanctioned or encouraged."

Using the Moos Family Environment Scale,[52] scores from the parents in 15 physically abusive families were compared with scores from the parents in 15 nonabusive families. The abusive families were less supportive of one another, less free to express their wants and desires, and less likely to have a common positive basis for family interaction than were nonabusive families. Abusive families were found to be more likely to express anger and aggression, more rigid in rule making and in structuring family activities, and more likely to be arranged in a hierarchical manner than nonabusive families.

General Observations and Studies

It is interesting to note that studies of physically abused children show that there is hardly ever a breakdown in the care of the child in other areas. They are usually fed, clean, and clothed well. The basic problem is with the mother's attitude. A breakdown has occurred in the natural emotional response of nurturing a child. Studies show that tension and disruption within the family unit occurs often during the act of feeding, cleaning, and comforting the child. The mother becomes upset and abuses her child.

A 1977 report in the *Journal of Pediatrics* [53] found no statistical differences in major psychological symptoms between abused and nonabused poor children. It was the general quality of parent/child relations, not the abuse/nonabuse dichotomy that produced the emotional differences in the children.

A California pilot study[54] on child abuse patterns revealed the following: If we include abused children of all ages, males predominate as the perpetrators of violence. If we select only children under three, females predominate significantly as perpetrators. Most violent incidents, with few exceptions, take place between September and February, and 59.3% of the injuries were inflicted by hand; 46.4% with an instrument; 5.6% as a result of kicking; 2.1% by strangling; 0.79% from stabbing; 10.7% from burning; 7.1% from direct neglect and exposure; and 4.3% from tying up. The percentage of non-life-threatening injuries was 71.5%.

Ray E. Helfer and C. Henry Kempe, in their study[55] *The Battered Child* (1968), state that "the number of children under five years of age killed by parents each year is higher than the number of those that die of disease." Studies also indicate that as many as 20% of all children seen in hospital emergency rooms may have injuries from either neglect or abuse.

Studies[56] show that abusive parents tend to be isolated in their environment. Many of these parents kept their blinds drawn on the house, even during bright, warm, sunny days. It was not uncommon to find within this group a higher percentage of unlisted phone numbers, for no apparent reason. There seemed to be more than the usual difficulty in maintaining automobiles, as well as a high frequency of breakdown of household appliances. These individuals, one would assume, were experiencing ego disorganization. Not only do they have a general fear of the world around them, but just as they are not able to pay enough attention to their children, they are unable to pay attention to their personal belongings.

Though one parent is usually the perpetrator of the attack on the infant, usually the mother, the other parent almost invariably contributes in some way, by accepting or even abetting it.[57,58] When questioned later, the nonabusing parent has known about such activity in the past and knows that family "pattern" of this abuse. The nonabusing parent will go through a familiar scenario again and again seemingly unaware of what will happen next. For example, a husband will demean and reject his wife and later that day she will abuse the child. Time and again, they will enact this tragic family drama. In homes where a child is abused, the mother will approach each task of infant care with three attitudes[59] that are usually in conflict with each other: (1) a desire to do something good for the infant; (2) yearning for the infant to respond to her and fulfill the emptiness in the mother's life in order to bolster her self-esteem; and (3) authoritative, punitive demands for the infant's correct response and behavior. If the caring task goes well, an attack on the child will not occur. But if anything interferes with the success of the parent's care, or increases the parent's feeling of being unloved, the punitive, harsh qualities will likely emerge.

Failure to Thrive[60,61]

"Failure to thrive" has had many definitions and designations: a child's growth failure, retardation, maternal deprivation syndrome, or deprivation dwarfism. The evidence that this illness has a psychological-sociological basis can be easily proved. Many of these children do poorly in foundling homes, orphanages, and other institutions, where they are raised. They often don't eat well or gain weight, appear depressed, withdrawn, with a flat affect. They become ill and often waste away—a condition sometimes called marasmus. This condition may be found in homes where the child is supposedly well taken care of. Yet there seems to be an inadequacy of basic nurturing for the infant with a lack of emotional warmth, physical contact, and sensory stimulation.

Failure to thrive (FTT) is now an established physiological growth disorder in which a child's weight is below the third percentile for his age. The child seems to obtain fewer calories or utilizes calories in a poorer way. There is no organic cause, and the etiology is centered on an omission of or disturbance in the parent/child relationship.

The problem is found in 3% to 5% of infants. Studies show that parents of FTT children invariably deny that there is any possibility of an interactional etiology for their child's malnutrition. They say that their children have no problems (52%), are "bad" (25%), or are physically ill (23%) in some unknown way. They deny that their children are not getting enough calories, even after physicians demonstrate plenty of evidence that the children are undernourished. The parents who have the most denial can actually convince themselves that the problem doesn't exist.

Characteristically, with these parents an emotional isolation between mother and child is usually the source of the problem. These parents do not readily play with their children, and tend to avoid any physical contact, even when the child is in distress. Clinical observation of the parents shows them as being manipulative and superficial (69%) or clearly depressed and over-whelmed by their life circumstances (31%).

The mothers of these children show early childhood distur-bances, and poor performances in current day-to-day activities. They tend to be dependent. Their thinking is concrete, though they rarely plan for the future and tend to use mechanisms of denial (saying something is not so that is), isolation (separating oneself or part of oneself from social interaction), and projection (ascribing to others one's own attitude, e.g., hostility). They are usually impulsive rather than careful planners. Their object rela-tions (emotional sharing and receiving from others in their childhood and into the present) were limited. Their feeling of identity is poor, so they have difficulty identifying in a positive way with their own infants. Their basic quality is a severe un-derlying depression; they literally live from day to day. Typ-ically, they had little mothering in their own childhood, and in their adolescence they gave up hope of ever receiving the nur-turing they so desperately needed.

When approached by males who offered some measure of friendship, or affection (no matter how superficial), intercourse and pregnancy with or without marriage is common. Usually, the inadequacy of the relationship is such that the person they selected will not be supportive enough. With the birth of a new child they are unable to cope without some external support. When they do not receive it they withdraw into their own de-pression and are unable to respond to the baby. The mother will avoid the infant, pay little attention to him, and give the child very little tactile stimulation (holding, stroking, soothing, cud-dling). Her reaction to the child is essentially mechanical.

When these children are brought to the hospital, they begin to improve even under the caring and loving ministrations of the nurses, student nurses, and nurses' aides. When the moth-ers come to feed the children, the nurses try to help the mother relate better to her child. Some of these sessions are observed (by hidden cameras) to discover how the mother usually feeds her child. Often the child will be lying in her lap with the bottle held mechanically in one hand and the mother smoking a cigarette with the other, or sometimes reading a book or magazine. There is no real interaction. Often when the child returns home he will lapse into his former debilitated state.

Sexual Abuse[C]

Research has shown that children are at a higher risk of sexual abuse when they live with a stepfather or mother's boyfriend, rather than with their natural fathers. Evidence also shows that as women become more secure—more assertive, less immature, and less childlike in their sexual roles—men who have doubts about their own adequacy may start to feel more threatened. As a result, they prefer the passivity and uncritical compliance of a sexual partner who is more childlike. Eventually, they may find a child more attractive as a sexual choice.

In a 1983 study[62] of sexual exploitation, younger women reported more intrafamilial sexual abuse than older women. This may be due to better recall or a greater willingness to report. However, the study found no comparable increase in extrafamilial abuse, indicating that there may have been an increase in intrafamilial sexual abuse over the past 30 years. The study also found that the vast preponderance of sexual abusers are males: men constitute 95% of the perpetrators of sexual abuse of girls, and 80% of the sexual abuse of boys. We can see, then, that physical abuse may be a problem of parenting (mothering); but sexual abuse seems to be a problem of masculine pathology.

A report in 1979[63] showed that nationally as many as 10% of boys and 20% of girls are victims of sexual abuse. A 1981 report of a sample of 583 sexually abused children indicated that 6% involved the father, 30% involved stepfathers, 15% involved other relatives, such as grandfathers, uncles, and brothers, and 6% were nonrelated parenting figures, such as the mother's boyfriend. Only 8% involved a stranger, and 35% involved an acquaintance of the child or the child's family.

Various studies of child molesters[64-69] have found that they are dependent, inadequate individuals with early histories characterized not only by conflict, but by disruption and abandonment. Often abuse and exploitation have been an integral part of their lives.

In 1979, Minnesota Multiphasic Personality Inventory (MMPI)[70,71] profiles were done of incestuous and nonincestuous child sex offenders. Many common features were found. They included feelings of insecurity and inadequacy in interpersonal relationships, dependency problems, and early family histories characterized by social isolation and family turmoil. The only difference between the two groups was that the nonincestuous offenders functioned at a lower level of sexual maturity. That is, the nonfamily child offenders were the most primitive in their psychological reactions.

David Finkelhor, in his study *Child Sexual Abuse*,[72] describes some of the social differences between men and women as follows:

1. Women learn earlier and much more completely to distinguish between sexual and nonsexual forms of affection.
2. Men grow up seeing heterosexual success—unrealistic proof that they are men—as much more important to their gender identities than women do. For example, having many sexual partners (conquests) is manly.
3. Men are socialized to be able to focus their sexual interest around sexual acts isolated from the context of a relationship.
4. Men are socialized to see as their appropriate sexual object persons who are younger and smaller than themselves, while women are socialized to see as their appropriate sexual partner persons older and larger.

As a result of the preceding information we can assume that men who are comfortable in relating to women at their same level of maturity and competence will be less likely to exploit children sexually. The opposite also holds true.

Both boys and girls are sexually abused, although girls are abused more often. The age range is primarily between 8 and 12 years old. In lower income families, girls are twice as likely to be sexually victimized than in the general population. However, in families with incomes over $20,000 (1980 dollars) with the ability to send children to college, 20% of the female victims are sexually abused in their childhood. A large percentage of children who grow up on farms are sexually victimized. It also seems that those girls who have fewer friends are much more vulnerable to sexual attacks. Of sexually abused girls with stepfathers, 50% are victimized by someone, not necessarily their stepfather. A stepfather is five times more likely to sexually victimize his stepdaughter than a natural father. Studies[73,74] have found that one out of six women with a stepfather as a principle figure in her childhood was sexually abused by him, compared to a rate of one of 40 for a biological father. Girls with stepfathers were five times more likely to be victimized by a friend of their parents.

When a father is particularly conservative, believing strongly in obedient children and the subordination of women, a daughter is more at risk. When he gives her little physical affection, this adds to the risk, because she hungers for affection, needs it, and may seek it from men who will abuse her. The presence of the mother is also an important factor. Girls who live without their natural mothers are three times more vulnerable to sexual abuse than the average girl. If the mother is emotionally distant or often ill, the girl is at higher risk, as well—not necessarily due to lack of supervision, since daughters of mothers who work are not at a higher risk. Rather, these girls require more affection than they are receiving.

When mothers are powerless victims in their own homes

and are controlled by their husbands, the incidence of sexual abuse of their daughters is higher. The more dangerous parental combination for a daughter is not when both parents are fully educated, but when the father is well educated and the mother is not. Again, it is the depreciation of the female that is usually the most significant factor.

Mothers of victimized girls are found to have been more punitive about sexual matters. These mothers would warn, scold, and punish their daughters for even asking questions about masturbation. The girl with a sexually punitive mother is 75% more vulnerable to sexual victimization than any typical girl in the study. This is the second most significant predictor of victimization. The first is having a stepfather. Thus, sexually rigid families, not those that are sexually lax, foster a high risk for sexual exploitation of female children.

It is interesting to note that there is little connection between physical abuse and sexual abuse. There is no other social variable that seems to be related to sexual abuse: religion, ethnicity, family size, or crowded quarters are not particular indicators. According to one major study there are eight independent predictors of sexual victimization: (1) the presence of a stepfather; (2) if the child ever lived without the mother; (3) if the child is not close to the mother; (4) if the mother never finished high school; (5) if the mother is sexually punitive (rigid); (6) if the father offers no normal physical affection to the daughter; (7) if the family has an income under $10,000 (1980 dollars); and (8) if the child has two friends or less during childhood. In those children with none of these factors present in their background, victimization is essentially nonexistent. Of those with five of these factors, two-thirds have been victimized. The presence, therefore, of each additional factor increases a child's vulnerability between 10% and 20%. This linear relationship can be graphed and is very dramatic.

In another study[75] the most common age for the sexual abuse of children was shown to be between 7 and 12. Another researcher found the mean age for girls was 10.2 and for boys only 7.2.[76]

In looking at other characteristics of the social structure of the female victims of sexual abuse, we find the following: lived on a farm, parents had an unhappy marriage, rigid family values, never finished high school, and mother still spanked the child at age 12.

Individuals who are sexual offenders do not seem to be motivated by sexual interest or desire: they are involved, rather, in a power struggle where they know that they can dominate the victim. In pedophilia (not forced rape), there is a strong erotic component that includes caressing and touching, although that is not possible until the power aspect of the relationship has been established. Child molesters are childlike themselves in their emotional needs, and have a need to relate to a child emotionally as being on a par with them. They generally have low self-esteem, and feel ineffective in adult social relationships. The sexual relationship with the child gives them the sense of power and control that they so desperately need. Some researchers have found more childhood sexual victimization in the backgrounds of sex abusers than in a variety of comparison groups.

Some psychoanalytic writers, in exploring the child molester, see him as having intense castration anxiety with a great fear of his mother as the castrator. If he is married he usually has a disturbed marital relationship, where the wife has become alienated. The husband (the molester) is too inhibited to find a solution to his marital problems and turns to his own or another's child instead. Some studies have shown that child molesters are among the most repressed of all sex offenders. They were reared by parents who were the least permissive regarding premarital and extramarital intercourse—an attitude which most molesters share with their parents.

Between 32 and 57% of child molesters reported some form of sexual trauma in their early development, compared to 3% of the general population.[77] Fortunately, most children who are molested do not go on to become molesters themselves. This is particularly true among women, who rarely become offenders, whether they were victimized or not.

David Finkelhor[78] set up as a model four preconditions for sexual abuse: (1) a potential offender needs to have some motivation to sexually abuse a child; (2) the potential offender has to overcome internal inhibitions against acting on that motivation; (3) the potential offender has to overcome external impediments to committing sexual abuse; and (4) the potential offender or some other factor has to undermine or overcome a child's possible resistance to the sexual abuse.

Certain aspects of the social environment early in the life of an abused child, as well as the cultural milieu in which the abuser operates, allow more possibility for sexual abuse to occur. For example, in a society that has a masculine requirement to be dominant and powerful in regard to sexual relations, sexual abuse is more likely to occur. This coincides with the male tendency to sexualize all of his emotional needs. There also seems to be an increase in child abuse relative to the increase in pornography available, particularly child pornography. Pornography seems to increase the legitimacy of this activity. It does not necessarily cause the abuse, but it lowers the judgment barriers for some individuals. It also indicates indirectly societal approval by its availability.

In a society where there is lack of social support for the mother, such as barriers to women's equality, abuse is more likely to occur. A mother who is not close to or protective of her child, or a mother who is dominated or abused by her husband, will also contribute to the problem. Further, the ideology of "family sanctity," which prevents external observance as a limitation of "family rights," allows such secret abuse to occur undetected.

If you add to the type of family situation, and society, (1) a child who is emotionally insecure and deprived searching for love, as well as (2) a situation of unusual trust between the child and the sexual offender, such as with a caretaker of the child, or a teacher, plus (3) today's society where a child is socially powerless, you have all the ingredients for sexual child abuse. Without a vote the child has no political clout. Legally it has little strength. Socially, culturally, religiously, advocacy is more for parental power and rights than those for children. Psychologically, economically, and intellectually, the child is even more powerless.

One of the findings of David Finkelhor[79] is that it does not matter what the motivation for the sexual abuse is: *If the potential offender is inhibited by strong social taboos and restrictions from acting, then abuse is highly unlikely to occur.* We should remember here that the prepubescent female holds a strong attraction to many adult males in our society who are sexually immature and would find difficulty in a relationship with a mature woman. They find it easier to approach and use a young girl.

What is there about a child that may lead to possible sexual abuse? If children are not under constant surveillance by their parents, if a child has a strong need for affection and is not getting it, the child may be more susceptible to sexual abuse. Thus, when we find a mother who is absent from the family because of divorce, death, or illness, her children tend to suffer more abuse. Also, if the mother is psychologically absent because of her serious emotional disturbance, a similar problem of increased sexual abuse may occur. It is also true that some children are sensed as making themselves "targets" while others are not. In a family of a few children, a father will select one child over another as a target because of that child's starvation for affection and its ability and need to respond. In a playground, one child will be selected more readily than another child as a target because somehow the child is communicating to the abuser in a nonverbal fashion that he will be susceptible to that attention. Some molesters can pick out victims from a public setting, such as a schoolyard. They have been quoted as saying that they "know" in an almost instinctual way who is a promising victim. It should be noted here that the child who seems suitable for abuse has been a victim long before the sexual abuse occurs.

The Appearance of the Abused Child[80,81]

The physically abused child does not always appear abused, since much of the physical injury may be covered by clothing. Sometimes, however, signs are visible that are not physical: (1) a small child who is more compliant than average; (2) child is negativistic; (3) seems unhappy; (4) is often angry; (5) seems isolated; (6) exhibits destructive behavior; (7) shows abusive behavior toward other children; (8) has difficulty developing relationships with other children; (9) shows excessive or complete absence of anxiety about being separated from parents; (10) shows inappropriate behavior toward parents, such as trying to take care of them; and (11) the child is constantly searching for attention and favors. In some developmental skills (cognition, language, fine and gross motor coordinations) there seem to be some developmental delays. Physical signs, other than actually finding the marks of physical abuse, would be malnutrition, pica (the craving to eat substances unfit for consumption, such as chalk or dirt), fatigue or listlessness, poor hygiene, and inadequate clothing. Some other obvious signs would be lack of appropriate adult supervision, a child repeatedly ingesting harmful substances (aspirin overdose), poor school attendance, a child who seems to be exploited and begs or steals (or is forced to), or a child who has excessive responsibilities at home. Many abused children show role reversal, where the child acts like a parental caretaker. Another indication is if the child begins using drugs or alcohol well before the teenage years.

In addition, the child may not get adequate medical attention or appropriate medical care if he has a serious or chronic illness; perhaps the child is not immunized, has inadequate dental care, or is not provided proper prosthetics, glasses, for instance.

The child who is sexually abused may: (1) confide in a relative or friend in some manner about the experience; (2) be withdrawn and have daydreams; (3) have poor peer relations; (4) show poor self-esteem; (5) appear phobic or anxious around adults; (6) have a distorted body image; (7) show shame or guilt; (8) show a sudden change or deterioration in academic performance; (9) exhibit a pseudo-mature personality; (10) make suicide threats or attempts; (11) have an excessively positive relationship with the offender; (12) be incontinent; (13) masturbate in an inappropriate manner more openly and excessively; (14) partake in highly sexualized play; and (15) hint about evidence in the family that another sibling has been sexually abused.

In an interesting study by Richard Galdston[82,83] done between 1968 and 1978, he observed 175 families with many children, including 100 families where an adult *seriously physically assaulted* a child. He looked primarily at the psychological factors involved. He found that though an abused child may cringe when his parents approach, he will cry and cling anxiously to them when they try to leave. Nevertheless, serious physical abuse is less serious a problem than primary neglect or deprivation.

A mind (ego) that is damaged in its early (0-5 years) development is almost beyond repair—i.e., psychotic, borderline psychotic, mentally retarded. This to me is more severe impairment than the physical crippling, as horrible as that is. There is also no doubt that a physically abused child will also be psychologically damaged. But, abandonment, coldness, and emotional neglect damages the mind the most. The emotional warmth of a loving mother (and family) available to the child is absolutely necessary for its normal mental development.

Galdston[84,85] sees neglect or deprivation as halfway between suicide and homicide. The abusing parent is tied to the child by the feeling that the child is actually persecuting her. She accuses the infant of crying deliberately to interrupt her sleep and believes that the toddler is maliciously trying to get into trouble.

Child abuse has been found to be a *family affair*. The same mothers who will be physically abusive to their children may be exemplary foster mothers, temporarily caring for other women's children. One of the women in Galdston's study was honored as the "Head Start Mother of the Year." It was only when she parented her own child that she dealt most intimately with the hated elements within herself and projected them onto her child. Thus, abuse of a small child almost always requires a domestic relationship.

Reading this material is far from comfortable. Though much of the detail and description of the physical abuse of children has been eliminated, our identification and empathy with these children is nonetheless painful. What then is even more difficult to come to terms with is the knowledge that this has been extant in the world for our entire recorded history and continues to the present. What may be even more difficult to assimilate is that abandonment (real and/or emotional) is *more injurious* to the child than sexual or physical abuse. A true understanding of this concept reveals my motivation in trying to understand "our ancestors."

Children perceive the world in a similar fashion, in all the world's history, for the first two years of their life; by three they are making more social perceptions beyond the immediate family; and, by five, are part of the local community. The organization of the first two years of life is fundamentally determined by the psychological health of the mother and the way the mother relates to the child; and the security, stability, and warmth of the immediate family unit. A child grows in the womb of the family, not only in the uterus of the mother.

In a society where women are respected, loved, and protected in the family, they are more likely to be healthy and not depressed; and thereby more likely to provide the appropriate nutrient love for the child. In a family that feels secure, an environment of security and love is likely to be provided to the mother and child.

Chapter 9

Conclusion: Our Future from the Past

Ad Astra per Aspera—To the Stars with Difficulty

We have traveled a long way—from Africa, to the Middle East, to Europe, to Asia and back again to North America. We have looked at the world as it was from 4000 B.C. to the present, and no matter where we have looked during our journey of 6000 years we have seen evidence of human violence toward children. It is written on papyri recovered from the tombs of ancient Egypt, in the Bible, carved on tombstones, and now is printed in the daily newspaper that is thrown each morning on our front steps. We are still killing and abusing our children. We are still devaluing family life. And today, in almost 2000 A.D., we are still denigrating women in our cultures.

We are living in a time that has seen still more space travel by man. Our skyscrapers are tall, our cities are modern, our tastes are sophisticated, and still our media deliver more news of this seemingly endless cycle of abuse.

A wire story just two paragraphs long blares this terrifying headline: (August 4, 1989) "20 Million Kids Reported Enslaved in South Asia." According to the article, these 20 million children are living in bonded slavery in South Asia, half of them in India—a report issued by the Anti-Slavery Society. A spokesman for the group speaking to the United Nations Commission on Human Rights commented: "This system is perpetuated in India and also in Pakistan, Nepal, Bangladesh, and Sri Lanka."

What have we learned? Perhaps more importantly, how can we apply what we have learned to understand this abuse and finally end it?

Sociologists who have studied the lopsided mortality rates that have existed throughout history tell us that when we see high rates of female mortality among young girls in a society, those rates may be a result of economic pressures on parents— especially those in an agrarian society who feel they need sons to work the land and who can only afford to feed a limited number of mouths within their family. But before we blame economic pressures, we have to understand that in these cases a cultural choice has also been made. Parents have chosen between sons and daughters, and they have found daughters to be less valuable.

Sociologists claim[1] that with the growth and development of manufacturing and large cities, the difference in perceived "value" between sons and daughters should have been eliminated. After all, child labor laws established an equal period of childhood for boys and girls, and with increased manufacturing there is now a job market for young women. Therefore, as a culture's standard of living rose, favoritism toward sons should not have remained. Yet these facts did not affect the female child mortality rates.

Personally, I find this view difficult to accept. As we have learned, child abuse—the most severe case being infanticide— has been prevalent in our world since people began recording history. Since that time there has always been more abuse and murder of girls than of boys. We cannot minimize the psychological and other sociological/ethnological factors that caused this imbalance.

As we have seen, numerous studies have pointed to individual, familial, and societal pathologies that exist when parents abuse or even kill their children. However, there is more to it than a bad economy. To find the real causes, whether historical or current, we have to look below the surface.

When abusive parents are tested (a superficial process), their psychological profile looks very much like that of the general population. However, certain differences can be noted in addition to those previously mentioned. (1) Their cognitive styles tend to be action oriented as opposed to depending more on thought and delaying impulse gratification. (2) They have strong oral dependent needs, with identity conflicts. (3) They have a strong defense against appearing depressed but, underlying, a significant depression exists. (4) They doubt their own adequacy as wives, mothers, husbands, and fathers. (5) Their ego identity is not age-appropriate.

According to Richard Galdston, in his study *Domestic Dimensions of Violence*,[2] we can look at abused children as part of the continuum of a dysfunction of the normal parenting process. This dysfunction has a continuum from neglect to deprivation, and from exploitation to abuse. Or child abuse can be seen as four different clinical entities. The first, "neglect," is a situation where the child is not cared for by the parent. The parent does not consider the child to have personal value and pays no attention to him. The neglected child is left to his own devices, with a variety of others raising him and functioning as surrogate parents. These parents are unable to perceive, recognize, or acknowledge that their child belongs to them, in any particular close relationship.

In the second category, "deprivation" of the child, the parents don't value the child as human. They acknowledge the child as their own, but not as a human being. This deprived child is usually raised in accordance with some bizarre ideas of how to toilet-train. For example, they must care for the child in some perverted way, such as rubbing the child's face in its feces, just as one might paper-train a dog. Educational methods may be instituted with a ruthless quality that does not recognize the child as a human entity. These parents deprive their child of human contact and don't recognize the child as being their biological issue, but rather as a vehicle for an idea or an object to employ in some particular way. Therefore, although these parents are not necessarily psychotic in any other area, they are psychotic in their relationship to their child. They may even give their child an outlandish nonhuman name such as Rover. These parents tend to have major compulsive constraints on their own behavior and tend to be rigid and disturbed in their contact with reality regarding the child. In other ways they fail to protect their child from real dangers.

In the third category, "exploitation," the parent uses the child to service his own needs and deal with his own appetites. This exploited child may develop specialized skills or be trained in a certain way. The child may be loved by the parents as human, but only because he is "useful." The child is usually precociously mature, with some early specialized adult quality. These children are caricatures of adults. As long as the child behaves in accordance with the parent's requirements, the parent/child relationship remains stable. However, when the child matures and no longer wishes to adhere to parental requirements, the relationship becomes explosive and dangerous.

In the fourth category, "physical abuse," there is a real physical assault upon a little child by the adult. (I have purposely not discussed here the physical abuse of teenagers. The abuse of a teen can be a continuation of a lifelong abuse of that child from the earliest years; or it can be a relatively new phenomenon related to teen/parental conflict that is on a different psychological basis than early childhood abuse. This is a long topic in itself and deserves a book of its own.) This differs from corporal punishment in that the child is too immature to understand he has committed a misdeed. The punishment not only is inappropriate in its severity but also in regard to the child's age.

A very young child cannot comprehend the message behind the punishment. This type of child abuse shows ambivalence in the parent's attitude toward the child. Between six months and three or four years of age, this child will characteristically have fresh and old bruises, welts and injuries, as well as fractures. Despite the abuse, the child will often be given special medical attention—repeated visits to clinics and to doctors—and the child will likely be well fed and well dressed. The child is both loved and hated by his parent at the same time.

Little boys who have been physically abused often develop a tendency toward violent behavior as their primary way of relating to other children. It is the main communication system they have learned from their parents. The parents, meanwhile, are unable to deal with their ambivalent feelings toward their child without resorting to some impulsive and violent discharge of emotions. Their view of the child is exaggerated in both extremes. The child is seen alternately as a saint and a sinner; a darling child and a "monster." Thus the parents vacillate rapidly between a highly inflated aspiration for the child and an inappropriate disappointment and hatred of the child—a roller-coaster response. They look to the child to confirm their position, and the attitude of punishment and discipline becomes obsessionally important to them. These parents are often not on reasonable terms with their own parents. Either they totally reject their parents or maintain a conflictual, intimate, immature tie to them while they are abusing their own child. They are also seriously depressed with an ego structure that is susceptible to psychotic disintegration, in other words, they could at any time completely lose touch with reality.

Family Study[3-5]

Studies of the parents who abuse children show that they have no more psychosis than usual population percentages. In other words, about 5% to 10% of the abusive parents are psychotic. There is obvious evidence of ego impairment in ordinary parenting qualities and child-rearing skills. These parents tend to be impulsive. They have a low tolerance of frustration, inadequate defenses (under minimal economic or social stress will become frightened, angry, and/or depressed), and foster a great deal of anger because they are frustrated over their inability to parent effectively. These parents exhibit evidence of a transference psychosis. They have a grossly distorted perception of their child; they attribute to the child hostile persecutory powers far beyond any semblance of reality. Aspects of the child/parent relationship are so distorted that the parent will have irrational fears and expectations regarding the child.

These same parents who abuse their children quite often have a great need even as adults to gain approval from their parents. Their marital and sexual histories are disturbed, often characterized by submission (passive/aggressive) and domination (masochism/sadism). It is not unusual for the abuse of the child to be a symptom of some disruption in the ordinary "balance of disharmony" in the marital relationship. Not only are there often chronic crises in the family unit, but at times of abuse there is usually an acute crisis of greater proportion—perhaps a change in jobs, finances, or physical moves. Central to this breakdown is the abusive parent's inability to maintain equilibrium.

Let us look for a moment at how the ego, the executive branch of the mind, operates. Karl Menninger's studies[6] of ego functioning produced some interesting and useful conclusions. His major concept was that the ego seeks homeostasis—steady state. This is achieved through a series of mental regulatory devices, which he divided into five orders or levels of ego functioning. If one level of ego function is not able to maintain homeostasis, the next lowest level will be used.

The first order is the least serious. In this level there is a conscious need to exert "will power" to master stress. This can lead to "hypersuppression or hyper-repression." The individual is irritable, hyperalert (almost "hyper" everything), shows reaction formation (an opposite reaction to the impulse), and/or has somatic symptoms.

The second order of regulatory devices of the ego shows a partial detachment from reality. The real world is at least partially decathected (less invested with feeling). Thus we find dissociation, phobias, magic substitutions, and substitution of self as an object for aggression—asceticism, self-mutilation, intoxication.

If the second order does not succeed, the ego will regress, in searching for homeostasis, to the third order (which is our prime concern). Here there is a "transitory ego rupture": the executive branch breaks down, characterized by violence, convulsions, panic, and extreme depression. All have the quality of episodic explosive outbursts of unorganized aggressive energy.

The fourth order is psychosis. And the fifth order is an irreversible reaction to stress, leading to death. (An example is the panic of someone lost in the woods exhausting themselves and dying of heart failure or of no known cause . . . "exposure.")

Within this framework the individual ego is viewed as seeking homeostasis and trying to stave off psychosis and death. Thus the aggressive outbursts of violent persons have a life-saving quality. They are a means of creating stability—the ultimate goal of the ego.

One of the most primitive human defenses is denial.[7] If an individual denies reality, he will not be able to cope with it. Eventually the challenges reality presents will overwhelm him. A primitive ego structure using a primitive psychological organization may handle the threat from reality by some aggressive primitive mode of expression—violence, for example.

Parents who beat their children will produce children who, when they become parents, will tend to beat their children. Parents who do not love, will not be able to teach their children to love. Parents who are not available will teach children to be parents who will not be available. Each generation will respond as it has been taught to respond. Only by increased understanding can parents reduce the repetition of their parents' behavior, and only with great effort. With effective psychotherapy more effective and useful understanding can be obtained. If the benefits can be available before their children are born (or soon thereafter) the chain of pathology from generation to generation (that incorrectly is seen as heredity) can be broken.

One of the common ways of living with your own destructive impulses is to deny that they are yours. Destruction then "originates" outside yourself and is perceived as being directed toward yourself: "It's not I; it is they." "It's the others who are causing the trouble." "It's the others who are provocative." Unconsciously, this is expressed by: "If they won't do it voluntarily, I will provoke them to provoke me." We find people who are provocative for the purpose of being provoked so they can retaliate and express their sadistic aggressive urges. All their behavior is rationalized to make the problem somebody else's, not their own.

An inability to cope with reality produces a state of psychic disequilibrium. Assuming there can be no change in the actual environment, the individual will have to make a change within himself; make an ego regression to try to seek equilibrium. Regression to a more primitive psychological level brings the person closer to the dangerous aggressive destructive impulses coming to the surface and, as a result, he will act violently.

The most important precursor for the production of violence in adults is early preschool exposure to violence, particularly in and by the family. If we view problem solving as an attempt to master the anxiety of having aggressive impulses, then the natural desire is to transpose oneself from the passive recipient of the situation to the active controller of it—from the passive beaten one to the active beater.

The battered child's parents have invariably been physically abused or repeatedly exposed to physical abuse during their own childhood. Those parents who do not batter their children, yet were themselves battered to a lesser degree, have the same need to hurt, though not as severely as their parents. Such parents may not come to the attention of the authorities as batterers. The controls they use may be the rigid control system of the primitive conscience. We know the rigid conscience works very well until it is overwhelmed by aggressive impulses. Then it falls apart. It is rigid, not flexible. Anything that causes these parents to have decreased controls is dangerous. Once they start to hit a child they may be unable to stop.

The danger in drugs, of which the worst is alcohol, is that they will affect the thinking parts of the brain first. This is no problem for most people, because they choose the times during which they will take this mild anesthetic. But if someone has poor ego control, a primitive psychological organization, he cannot afford to lose control. Therefore, sedative drugs of all kinds, particularly alcohol, are dangerous, and the poorer the psychological (ego) organization, the greater the danger.

Therese Benedek noted, in *Parenthood as a Development Phase*,[8] that childhood memories return when an adult becomes a parent. The memories return in two forms: (1) Adults remember what it is like to be a child, as well as (2) how they experienced being parented. Unconsciously, it is as if they cannot escape the cycle, they must "do unto their children as they were done unto." The mothers of abused children did not have a symbiotic, confidence-producing relationship with their mothers, and they repeat this with their own children.

By three months of age, the infant begins to lose his undifferentiated awareness of the world and gains a differentiated awareness of itself as separate from the object world. The "I" and the "non-I" are beginning. Thus, mother begins to become a pleasure-giving and frustration-producing object. The amount of giving and frustration the child experiences at this period will determine the child's basic self-concepts and its concept of mothering. The unresolved ambivalence of the giving and frustrating mother is typical of the parents of the abused child.

Both Benedek[9] and Erik Erikson[10] have written about this phenomenon, calling it "a basic trust in mother." The abusing parents did not have this confidence-producing experience in their childhood. When we examine the relationships of the abusing parent, we find they have "lots of good friends," but actually these are more acquaintances than close, real friends. Their "good friend" relationships are distant, superficial, and unfulfilling. Their social lives are relatively limited and isolated, though they have many contacts. Analysis shows that this is the result of a persistent pattern—the same lack of confidence they had in childhood with their parents, particularly their mother.

The early conscience of the child is developed by the responses of the frustrated parent. Children who have been abused, have a history (a history their parents share) of being told "no" early after birth—"no" in terms of "do this" and "don't do that," slapping, yanking, and making the infant obey, whether the child is being fed, diapered, or bathed. The child is made to be quiet and lie still by angry tones, blows, and jerking. If the child cries and doesn't respond to being comforted, the child becomes an accuser of the parent—a threat to the adult with the learned lack of confidence. Anything may be done then to protect the parent from such a threat.

Children identify early with their parents, even the ambivalent ones, and by so doing, establish a conscience that is not only harsh and punitive but also quite ambivalent. This primordial identification with the aggressor that begins in the early months of life is reinforced through the rest of the child's development into his second and third year. The child then has a true identification with the aggressor that he cannot escape. The child turns the aggression against himself as he grows older, and then reprojects the aggression onto his own children. This accounts for the depression, the feelings of inferiority, low self-esteem, and the marked ambivalence in parents who abuse.

Their earliest memories usually are of fighting between parents, whether this is a true or a screen memory. And they find it reprehensible when their child does not show "proper respect for authority," which, in their opinion, always warrants severe punishment. Abusive parents[11-13] use this "lack of respect" as righteous justification for their attitude toward their children. In testing the abusive parent, we find that they have basically early childhood (0-2 years) dependency/independency hedonistic conflicts, depression, a sense of worthlessness, and a poor self-concept.

Psychological profiles indicate successive generational disruptions of mothering. Brandt F. Steele and Carl B. Pollack, in their study *A Psychiatric Study of Parents Who Abuse Infants and Small Children*,[14] observe that punishment is the abusing parent's investment in the child. They punish the child in an attempt to change the child's behavior so as not to neglect the parent (undoing what happened to them).

Other studies[15] have noted three clusters of personality characteristics in the abusing parent. In the first category are parents burdened with a pervasive, poorly controlled hostility. Parents in the second category are rigid, compulsive, and lack warmth (coldness with little overt hostility). Parents in the third category are very depressed and unresponsive and appear passive and dependent, competing with the child for the spouse's attention.

A fourth category (occurring more frequently) consists of abusing fathers who are young, intelligent, have skills, but are unable to support their families. As a result, the wife has to work and the father stays home with the children. In his frustration, and because of his low self-esteem, he abuses the child for "not behaving."

Many studies[16-22] have shown that the child-abusing family has other elements of family dysfunction. Some authors have noted that there is a chronic state of anxiety as well as masochistic, self-destructive behavior in the parents, with a preoccupation and focus on external problems as being the constant danger, and an intense need to master the moment.

Pollack and Steele[23] tell us: "There seems to be an unbroken spectrum of parental action toward children ranging from the breaking of bones and fracturing of skulls through severe bruising to severe spanking and on to mild reminder pats on the bottom. To be aware of this, one has only to look at the families of one's friends and neighbors, to look and listen to the parent-child interactions at the playground, supermarket, or even recall how one raised one's own children or how one was raised one's self. The amount of yelling, scolding, slapping, punching, hitting, and yanking, acted out by parents on very small children is almost shocking. Hence we have felt that in dealing with the abused child we are not observing an isolated, unique phenomenon, but only the extreme form of what we would call a pattern or style of child rearing quite prevalent in our culture."

We find the same things in cultures of the ancient past as well. Sometimes it is easier to see a pathological process when we look at an extreme case of the problem in question. Earlier in this century, the severe lobar pneumonia ending in death gave medical scientists an understanding of that illness that they were unable to obtain from much milder benign respiratory infections. With this in mind, we will look at each society and see when things were at their worst for children. Then we can see what there was about that society, at that time, that contributed to the abuse. We can also do the reverse, and examine these same societies when things were much better for children.

Worst Situation

Up until Egypt became a militaristic country it treated its children kindly. But as war became more prevalent, family life broke down. The number of incestuous marriages increased, and the adequate care of children decreased. With the advent of the New Kingdom (1554-1075 B.C.) the Greeks began playing a greater role in the Egyptian community and Grecian philosophy infiltrated the Egyptian social structure. This increased when the Ptolemaic dynasty began and with that period came a marked decrease in the status of women. Gradually, there was also more evidence of slavery. In fact, slavery increased from the time of Ramses II, and grew particularly prevalent during the Ptolemaic period. Remembering then what we have learned, as the status of women declined, the psychological education of the child changed as well. Add to that increased slavery and you have an atmosphere in which children learned to be violent, learned to despise others, and ultimately learned to be abusive parents.

The most violent time for Hebrew children was during the biblical period of rigid patriarchy. This was the period of the *Lex Talionis* principle, when the attitude of the Hebrew people was harsher and less humane than at any other time in their history. During this period the Hebrews were more warlike than they would later become. They showed less affection toward women. New and foreign religious beliefs were introduced. Slavery was common and there was a distinct class system. It was at this time in their history that the Hebrews sacrificed children and abused them, however abnormal this was for the culture in later years.

The Greeks supported the most violence against infants and children when they were warlike. In fact, the most warlike among the Greeks, the Spartans, had the most severe, destructive attitude toward children. They trained them to be violent soldiers. The Greeks were brutal to their slaves and serfs. During the time of Pericles in later Athenian culture, the status of women decreased markedly and many freedoms were taken away. Slavery was increased, the courts became corrupted, family life was disrupted, and children died increasingly as a result.

Rome was the least abusive to its children *prior* to the onset of the empire, with its tyrannies and extensive conquests. The more they conquered, the more they destroyed their own children. As slavery increased, so did the level of family disruption. The courts became more and more corrupt and wars were incessant. As these social characteristics mounted the value of human life dropped, particularly for children.

In China's earliest period, prior to 220 B.C., less respect was given to human life than later on. Children received the harshest treatment during times of famine, plague, starvation, and particularly, during the period known as the Warring States (403-221 B.C.), when the general cultural patterns were disregarded and children were killed so that others could live and eat. However, the Chinese were never as severe in their disregard for human life as the Greeks and Romans were in the latter period of their development. The Yuan period (1260-1368 A.D.) began cultivating harsher attitudes in the community as the Chinese absorbed some of the Mongol and Tartar attitudes, which included infanticide. With the Ming restoration a puritanical attitude took hold that justified the Mongol harshness. Though harsher attitudes toward children prevailed, they still were treated relatively well. The worst period for child care in China was during the Ching (Manchu) dynasty (1644-1912 A.D.) when there were the greatest number of child slaves in Chinese society. Infanticide is recurring today under the Communists, who are penalizing families with more than one child. Often, if the firstborn is a girl, the child is killed to make way for a boy.

Best Situation

The best situation for children in Egypt was from its early dynastic period to the time of the Hyksos. The family was intact, few incestuous relationships existed, and large families were encouraged. Children remained close to their mothers during the first three years of life and were treated with care and respect.

The best period for the Hebrew children occurred following the second Diaspora and the post-Talmudic period when, following the precepts of the Talmud, the Jews began to honor both mother and child and put them first within their lives. Education was stressed in their society even more, and family cohesiveness increased. They became the least warlike in their entire history, and were no longer a nation with an army. They were at peace with themselves and with their children.

The most benign period for children in Greek society was prior to their becoming involved in extensive internecine warfare. When slavery was at a minimum in the land there was also greater freedom and respect for women. This was the period of the least infanticide and other forms of child abuse.

Rome had its most benign period when the family was central and important. In the days of kingship, clans were vital, and in postkingship times a republic and a relative democracy prevailed. Prior to their quest for an empire, the Romans showed a benign attitude to their children, to families, and to women. There was greater equality. Also, much less slavery existed.

The most benign period for children in China was from post-Chin 220 B.C. on until the onset of the Mongols in the 1300s. Except for episodes of famine, this ancient period of China was the most benign for almost 1500 years in its care for children. Families were mostly intact, the environment was consistent, little slavery was practiced, and women and sex were not depreciated. Children, then, saw by example the concepts of honoring one's parents and respecting life, and they carried those attitudes on in their own families.

As has been noted, there seems to be a historical relationship between slavery and other forms of human depreciation, child abuse, and infanticide. A historical correlation also seems to exist between the status of women in society and the amount of child abuse and infanticide. Furthermore, there seems to be a connection between the intactness and loving quality of a family relationship and the absence of child abuse. Essentially the more tyrannical and disrupted the family, particularly the latter, the more child abuse and infanticide will occur.

Three features characterize cultures and families where there is no child abuse. They have (1) stable marriages, (2) marital and family love, and (3) family and marital cooperation—that is, men, women, and children work together for the good of the family unit. The first and third items are characteristic of the ancient cultures of the Hebrews and the Chinese. The second quality, marital and family love, existed, but was not as extensive as the stability and cooperation in a family unit. In general we find more parental tenderness in the early Egyptian, Chinese, and Hebrew cultures. The more wars and separations of husbands from wives and fathers from sons, the more abuse in a society (compare chapters on Greece and Rome).

The Chinese and Hebrews promoted family and marital harmony. Furthermore, less maternal depression was found in these two cultures since women were less depreciated in China and among the Hebrews. In Egypt we find a much more positive response to women prior to the Ptolemies.

Few premature demands were placed upon children (1) in China, (2) by the Hebrews, and (3) in most of ancient Egypt; while this was not the case in Greece and Rome.

The stable, secure, homogeneous societies of early Egypt, the Hebrews, and China tended to produce more parental security, thus countering the parental insecurity that was often the precursor of child abuse. Insecure parents tend to take out their misery on their children.

Except during famine periods in China, children were not seen as the cause of any family difficulty: quite the opposite. This was also true in Egypt and among the Hebrews, but not in Greece and Rome, where parental whims came first and the needs of children were often never met. Later, in the West, this was carried on in the religious concepts of a child being related to "original sin," "corruption," and "wickedness."

Though there is an exceptional demand for premature child obedience in child-abusing families, and we see this both in China and in the West, in China there was a modifying factor of father's responsibility to his son, with clan supervision of the father. Conditions were similar among the Hebrews and in the early half of the Egyptian civilization.

Historically, we see that disrupted or inadequate mothering is an important factor in child abuse. We see it especially among the Greeks and Romans and less in early Egypt, among the Hebrews, and among the families in China.

Abusing families have always tended to be asocial or withdrawn. We find in most cultures that men tend to socialize without their wives outside the home. However, in China the parents socialize extensively within the family compound. The Hebrews also had a central organization of religion within the homes and wives played a primary role. Though there was religion in the homes of early Grecian and Roman families, this was not the case as these civilizations rose in economic and militaristic might; when the power of the empire increased women were accordingly depreciated, and there was less involvement in the home situation. This may have contributed to their high rate of child abuse and infanticide.

Parental and societal hostility was marked in Egypt following the expulsion of the Hyksos, among the Greeks and Romans, and in the early biblical period of the Hebrews. Other periods of these cultures saw less militarism, less hostility, and also less child abuse.

We find that the overstressed importance of authority is another characteristic of child abuse. All five cultures made a point of this. However, China modified the severity of this authority with the father/son identification. The Hebrews modified it significantly as they reached the Talmudic period. One of the characteristics of child-abusing families is that the parents who abuse their children have a very poor relationship with their own parents. This was highly unlikely for the Chinese, the Hebrews, and the Egyptians, who were intimately involved with their parents in a positive manner.

In child-abusing families the child is taught one way or another that the world is a dangerous place and the only safety lies in being frightened of the world and clinging to the family, no matter how abusive it is. This has been common instruction in the West, particularly among those successful warlike nations such as Sparta and Macedon. The Chinese child was taught that the family was stable and secure and that they were safe within it and the clan. They were also taught that China was the center of the universe and the rest of the world was relatively barbaric. Therefore they had a small-scale and large-scale environment to which they could relate. The Hebrews were taught to love the world, as all the world was part of God's creation, and all men were equal.

Abused children often have a history of some distortion in the weaning process. Current studies show that early weaners are more prone to abuse than late weaners because mothers who cease nursing early are cutting off some of the intimacy of their early relationship with the child. This was never the case in China, frequently the case in Greece and Rome, and less so in Egypt and among the Hebrews.

As everyone knows, it is very difficult to give yourself an injection. Diabetics have to be trained so that they can overcome resistance to hurting themselves. Even though they intellectually know it is to help themselves, they initially have to "steel their nerves" so that they can puncture their own skin. Often people have to force themselves to do "unnatural" things in order to take proper care of themselves. It is very hard to consciously hurt yourself. When we come across people who hurt themselves willingly we know that they are emotionally ill, and that they have a significant and serious problem.

It is obvious that if you see your children as an extension of yourself, it would be very difficult to inflict harm upon them. It is only when you hate and reject yourself, that you can come to hurt your own children. This pattern was not necessarily true of China. The Chinese culture was built on family. People cared for themselves and their families and developed close ties and identifications within the family unit. A unique relationship existed, particularly between father and son. This identification, not without its obvious ambivalence, produced a culture that was less abusive to its children than any other large culture in the West.

Further, it should be recognized in looking back over the literature on child-abuse patterns in the family, that a society that encourages violence gives more support to parents to be violent; thus adding to the vicious cycle that goes from generation to generation. In addition, a society that encourages in any way separation of mother and child in the early years of life is going to make it extremely difficult for that child to be secure and have a solid identification with an individual, particularly someone who is motherly. This was found in the early years of the new State of Israel, when children raised in a kibbutz nursery had significant psychological problems when they grew to adulthood. This propelled a change in this aspect of the kibbutz child rearing, with less separation of mother and child (see Bruno Bettelheim, *Children of the Dream*).[26]

A cohesive society that is kind to its children, has a certain homogeneity, and family togetherness, and avoids separation of mother and child, will raise its children to continue that society's culture, a culture of kindness to children.

However, if it is a culture of hatred, aggression, rejection of children, separation of mother and child, depreciation of mothers and women, will not those children tend to hate and reject themselves, particularly as they identify with aggressive, punitive, and ambivalently perceived parents? As adults, won't those former children form a society full of self-haters and self-rejecters? Won't a society that hates and rejects itself or members of its society have a higher percentage of child abusers and abusers of other members of the society? Is it not also more likely to become a society that is aggressive outside its own borders? When there is not an external war, is it not more likely to turn its hostility against itself, often by hurting its own children?

It is true in the West that there is less abuse of children than there used to be. It is true that in this less-than-perfect society, conditions are getting better. But, is it not also true that we can learn from history that the abuse of children in the West is part and parcel of an erratic, unstable society, a society that has aggression, rigidity, separation of mother and child, and depreciation of children and women as major elements?

There was less abuse of children in the history of China than in most other societies. China also had more family and society continuity. It also had much less separation of mother and child and much less encouragement and support of aggression as a way of solving problems. In addition, it significantly encouraged a close father/son relationship. It stressed the importance of mothers as caregivers, and it stressed the importance of education far beyond that in the ancient West. In the West, support and encouragement was given to the hostility of the fighter. This was rarely the case in China.

It is also true that the Hebrews, despite their small numbers, and despite their gross dispersion into the wider Diaspora, maintained (even more so than the Chinese) a continuity, a cohesiveness, a family togetherness and, obviously, much less child abuse than any other segment of society in history. It was a society that is fundamentally based on peace and freedom. It was one that stressed the importance of mothers and the love of one's fellow man.

We see, therefore, the patterns—not scant, not isolated, but real patterns in cultures that lead the people of that culture to or away from child abuse. What, then, do we do about it?

Recommendations[24]

In 1985 a sociological study was done of 45 abusing families. Few (25%) showed any noticeable improvement in child care while receiving services from the Public Child Welfare Agency that offered little if any psychotherapy. Many families, in fact, deteriorated even further. The deprivation was never dealt with. Researchers found that a substantial proportion of America's children were living in families that lacked what most Americans considered essential conditions for growing up healthy without fear and pain. Therefore, they made various recommendations:

1. A homemaker service is crucial to prevent further child abuse and neglect. The service will provide a necessary respite for the mother as well as another adult to whom she can relate. This is especially useful when cooperation of other adults who might live in the home is scarce.

2. Day care should be used as a means of modifying the problem of child abuse. Although the quality of day care is important, it can never compare to the care of a mother caring for her child at home. If the day care is consistent and not overused it can help modify the problem.

3. Some kind of economic assistance, in the form of jobs for members of the family unit, should be provided. These jobs should offer some measure of self-respect as well as monetary gain.

4. Birth planning programs, where money is supplied through Medicaid and other state sources for procedures such as abortions, vasectomies, tubal ligations, and other forms of contraception, should be provided.

5. The establishment of alcohol treatment programs is necessary, since alcohol abuse is an extensive contributor to the problem of child abuse. (Unfortunately, the report left out the

most important service, namely psychotherapy. As long as the services offered are external props and do not deal with the intrafamilial and individual psychological problems, the benefits will be very limited.)

Their general conclusion was as follows:

"Economic factors affect the level of personal resources, and therefore the importance of social resources for successful parenthood. Poor people generally have fewer personal resources, and thus their need for social resources is greater if they are to succeed as parents. Rich people generally have more personal resources, and therefore they are less dependent upon social resources. For this reason the importance of the neighborhood varies as a function of economic resources. Rich people can better afford a weak neighborhood then can poor people, who must rely much more heavily on the social resources of their ecological niche for support, encouragement, and feedback." Simply put, where there is stress on the family—and this was true of the ancients as well as it is today—child abuse is more likely to take place. Economic stress makes it more difficult to function, can hurt family unity, and therefore, can lead to family violence.

David Gil,[25] in his 1970 book *Violence against Children: Physical Child Abuse in the United States*, states that much child abuse is related to distortions in social policies and general public practices. "The abuse of children is human originated acts of commission or omission and human created or tolerated conditions that inhibit or preclude unfolding in development of inherent potential of children. . . .

"Children have few acknowledged rights and they are not regarded or respected and treated as persons in their own right. Rather they are perceived as objects belonging to their parents or other adults. . . .

"Study after study of reported incidence of child abuse has revealed a significant association between maltreatment of children and conditions of poverty reflected in unemployment, inadequate income, dependence on public assistance, substandard housing and neighborhoods, and similar factors. . . .

"Prevention of child abuse requires redefinitions of childhood and the rights and status of children in accordance with egalitarian and humanistic values. Children would have to be viewed as persons in their own right rather than rightless objects or property controlled by adults. Such redefinitions would involve categorical rejection of physical punishment and coercion in child rearing at home and in the public domain, and replacement of these violent and destructive measures with constructive, educational ones which convey respect and caring for children as individual human beings." Gil concludes by stating that "social transformation toward a nonviolent social order will not be an event, but an extended process initiated and carried out by political movements committed to these goals. Prevention of child abuse is therefore also a gradual process, since it is predicated on the transformation of the prevailing, violent social order in which it is a symptom, into a genuinely nonviolent order. Accordingly, prevention of child abuse as part of the political process involves a long series of steps, each of which needs to challenge elements of the violent social order associated with this destructive phenomenon: social values, definitions of childhood and children's rights, and institutional arrangements such as poverty and the organization of work and production which result in insecurity, frustration, and stress."

Provide a child with the same mothering figure for the first years of life—a mother who herself feels loved and lovable, and she will be more likely to provide that child with a loving environment. The child will experience adequate ego growth, feel lovable, identify with a parent who gives him a positive view about life, and will therefore be able to love others. The immediate family, if it is cohesive and secure, will more likely provide an extension of mother through which the child can grow. This benign family will, through identification, enable the child to work through the complexities of the fundamentals of human relationships (oedipal complex).

Families have choices to make. It is unquestionably true that men and women are equal. They deserve equal pay, equal respect, and equal freedom to live their lives as they wish. However, if together a man and woman decide to have children, and they want their child to grow up under the best circumstances, they must create a family atmosphere. How they will create and shape their family unity will determine, to a large degree, how successful their child will be. The child's future is in their hands. A woman who gives birth and then hands over her child to someone else to take care of must know that this decision will dramatically affect her child's future. Unfortunately, economic necessity sometimes determines that both husband and wife must work during the important formative years of their children's lives. Still, there are choices. Child care, then, is best handled within the home, with a consistent loving figure always available for the child's needs. It should be kept in mind that if the mother is disturbed or distressed, if she is required to be home with her child, it could be less traumatic for the child to have an additional caregiver for the child so the mother can get away or go to her preferred activities.

These may not be easy choices for men or women to make. But they are real issues and they must be addressed. Women and men are equally important. When they marry and decide to have children they must discuss who will care for the infant. It is their choice to make. If the wife chooses to be the primary breadwinner, then the husband must be the primary parent figure for the children and stay home to raise them. Usually the husband is chosen to be the primary breadwinner. If both choose to be breadwinners and leave the mothering of their children to another adult, that decision will ultimately have deleterious effects, as we have indicated.

We know that a girl who feels loved in a secure family relationship, is more likely to mature into a woman who can identify with her mother, and raise her own children in a loving way. She will be capable of identifying in a nonconflictual way with her child, and love this extension of herself. If this same girl is able to respect and love her body (especially her genitals), and appreciate her central importance in sexual activity and family continuity, then her body ego, gender/role identity, and self-respect will be healthier. She will also have fewer conflicts of unresolved hostility toward her parents. When such a girl matures and becomes a mother, she will not abuse her children or abandon them overtly, or covertly by rejection. This can only occur in a society that respects, values, and loves women and which strives to enhance family stability and security.

Fathers need a direct and early involvement with both sons and daughters in a positive way. It is necessary for the child's development and identity, as well as understanding the vital relationship that males have with their children and wives. This enables a child not only to establish its own gender role, but to understand and work through the complexities of a male/female relationship.

The successful development of a child has little to do with the economic level of that community or nation, as long as it is adequate for a healthy life. If there is family continuity, there is likely to be family security. If there is family security there is likely to be respect for its members. With mutual respect in a family, love will grow. Where there is love in a family, the mother will be loved. When the mother is loved, she is much more likely to love her children. When the children are loved, they are likely to grow up in a healthy way, and have healthy families themselves when they mature. Because of their identification with a loving object, and feeling lovable, children will be healthier. A community or a nation of healthy families with healthy children will not have a pattern of child abuse.

Those societies that have stressed (1) the importance of family, (2) mothers who are loving and equal to fathers in family importance, (3) love of children, (4) continuity of families and children, (5) the value of sexuality, (6) the importance of children's education, (7) the care for the elderly and the infirm, (8) the proper mourning for family loss, (9) the avoidance of separation of mother and child, (10) the stress of intellect over arms, and (11) respect for law will more likely produce a society of great continuity and strength and have little or no child abuse.

In the United States, approximately $2 billion is spent annually to treat about 0.5 million children who are in various foster care systems. Providing all families with a job that gives them some self-esteem might be a better way of spending that $2 billion and can help avoid the abuse and neglect in the first place. It also should be made part of public policy that corporal punishment and physical coercion of children in the public domain is forbidden by law. Cultural sanctions ought to be developed against such punishments and coercion in the private domain, as well. We have learned too well that these practices only hurt children—if not physically, then emotionally and developmentally.

Whatever resources and energies can be devoted to (1) enhancing the security of fathers in a home, (2) family stability, (3) the value of women (as equal to if not superior to men), and (4) the necessity of giving extensively to children in their most early formative years is vital. The more funds and resources we devote to the young family with its young children, the more benefits will be reaped for all of society in the next 20 to 40 years.

It is hard not to abuse others if you hate yourself. It is hard to abuse a child if you love yourself. But we cannot begin to love ourselves without changing our attitudes about the ultimate importance of family life, our children and the mothers who give them life. Nor can we hope that they will love themselves without our support.

When all is said and done, the most important person in our universe is the mother who can pass along her love, nurturing, security, and stability to her daughters, who will continue the cycle and pass along these characteristics to her children.

The preparation for motherhood begins in infancy. Without this foundation in the first two to three years of life, the little girl will become impaired in her functioning as a mother. This means that *the most important person in the world is a newborn female child*. What a horrible tragedy that she has been the object, throughout history, of society's prejudice and abuse. Without that love from mother we flounder; without it, there is pain, violence, death—even war. The only hope our civilization has lies in changing our response toward women. They should not be treated as equal to men; they deserve better.

"We learn best what our hearts prepare us to learn."

References

Chapter 1. Introduction

A. The extensive historical literature has been summarized. However, there are particular resources on the history of childhood that I have utilized in this Introduction. Therefore, I have included the following list as of specific interest. Particular attention should be given to the material by Aries and deMause.

Aries, P. 1965. *Centuries of Childhood: A Social History of Life*. New York: Vintage Books.

Becker, H. and R. Hill, eds. 1955. *Family, Marriages and Parenthood*. Boston: D. C. Heath Company.

Benedict, R. 1946. *Patterns of Culture*. New York: Penguin Press.

Boas, F. 1938. *General Anthropology*. Boston: D. C. Heath Company.

Caldwell, W. E. 1937. *The Ancient World*. New York: Rinehart.

DeBurgh, W. G. 1924. *The Legacy of the Ancient World*. New York: Macmillan.

deMause, L. ed. 1974. *The History of Childhood*. New York: Psychohistory Press.

deMause, L. 1974. *The Evolution of Childhood*. New York: Psychohistory Press.

Despert, J. 1965. *The Emotionally Disturbed Child: Then and Now*. New York: Brunner/Mazel.

Dunn, C. 1920. *The Natural History of the Child*. New York: John Layne Publisher, 308.

Ende, A. *Children in History*. New York: *Journal of Psychohistory*, 11:1.

Eyben, M. 1980. *Family Planning in Greco-Roman Antiquity, Ancient Society*. 11/12: 5-82.

Flandrin, J., 1979. *Families in Former Times: Kinship, Household and Sexuality*, Translated R. Southern. Cambridge, England: Cambridge University Press.

Garrison, F. H. 1965. *Abt-Garrison History of Pediatrics, Pediatrics*. Philadelphia: Saunders Co. Vol. 1.

Goodsell, W. 1934. *The History of Marriage and the Family*. New York: Macmillan.

Harris, M. 1977. *Cannibals and Kings: The Origins of Cultures*. New York: Random House.

Kramer, S. N. 1956. *From the Tablets of Sumer: 25 Firsts on Man's Recorded History*. Indian Hills, Colo: Falcons Wing Pub.

Langer, W. L. 1974. *Infanticide: A Historical Survey, History of Childhood Quarterly*. 1(3): 353-365.

McKee, L. 1982. *Preferential Care and Child Mortality Differentials*, Symposium on Indirect Infanticide & Sex Differentials in Children's Treatment, 81st Annual Meeting American Anthropological Assoc. Washington, D.C., Dec. 3-7, 1982.

Miller, B. D. 1981. *The Endangered Sex*. Ithaca, New York: Cornell University Press.

Nash, A. S. 1955. *Ancient Past and Living Present, Family Marriage and Parenthood*. Becker & Hill, 84-103.

Neel, J. V. 1970. *Lessons From A Primitive People, Science* 170, (3960): 815-822.

Payne, G. H. 1916. *The Child and Human Progress*. New York: G. B. Putnam Sons.

Pieper, A. 1966. *Chronik Kinderheilkunde, Veb Georg Thiem—History of Childhood*, Leipzig.

Radbill, S. X. 1968. *The Battered Child*, eds Helfer and Kempe. Chicago: University of Chicago Press.

Ruhrah, J. 1925. *Pediatrics of the Past*. New York: P. B. Holber.

Rush, F. 1981. *The Best Kept Secret: Sexual Abuse of Children*. New York: McGraw-Hill.

Ryan, W. B. 1862. *Infanticide: Its Law, Prevalence, Prevention and History*. London, England: J. Churchhill.

Seltman, C. 1956. *Women in Antiquity*. London—New York: Thames & Hudson.

Shiner, L. E. 1980. *The Darker Side of Hellas: Sexuality & Violence in Ancient Greece, Psychohistory Review*, 9(2).

Smith, P. 1934. *A History of Modern Culture*. New York: Vol. 2.

Trexler, R. 1973. *Infanticide, In Florence: New Sources and First Results, A History of Childhood Quarterly*, 1:98-116.

Vallois, H. V., 1961. *The Social Life of Early Man: The Evidence of Skeletons*. Chicago: University of Chicago Press.

Westermarck, E. 1921. *The History of Marriage*. London: Macmillan.

1. Bledsoe, C. H. 1983. *Stealing Food as a Problem in Demography and Nutrition*, Paper presented to 82nd Annual Meeting American Anthropological Association, Chicago, Nov. 16-10.
2. Balikci, A. 1967. *Female Infanticide on the Arctic Coast, Man*, 2: 615-625.
3. Birdsell, J. B. 1969. *Some Predictions for the Pleistocene Based on Equilibrium Systems Among the Hunter Gatherers, Man the Hunter*, Lee & Devore, eds. Chicago: Aldine, 229-240.
4. Boas, F. 1938. *General Anthropology*. Boston: D. C. Heath.
5. Dickeman, M. 1975. *Demographic Consequences of Infanticide in Man, Annual Review of Ecology and Systematics*, 6:107-137.
6. Goldman, I. 1970. *Ancient Polynesian Society*. Chicago: Chicago University Press.
7. Lipin, L. A. 1960. *The Assyrian Family in the Second Half of the Second Millennium B.C., Journal of World History*, 6: 628-643.
8. Pakrasi, K. 1970. *Female Infanticide in India*. Calcutta: Editions Indian.
9. Vallois, H. V. 1961. *The Social Life of Early Man: The Evidence of Skeletons*. Chicago: University of Chicago Press.
10. Ibid.
11. Eyben, M. 1980. *Family Planning in Greco-Roman Antiquity, Ancient Society*, 11/12: 5-82.
12. Balikci, A. 1967. *Female Infanticide on the Arctic Coast, Man*, 2: 615-625.
13. Birdsell, J. B. 1969. *Some Predictions*.
14. Boas, F. 1938. *General*.
15. Goldman, I. 1970. *Ancient Polynesian Society*. Chicago: Chicago University Press.
16. Pakrasi, K. 1970. *Female Infanticide in India*. Calcutta: Editions Indian.
17. Vallois, H. V. 1961. *The Social Life*.
18. Williamson, L. 1971. *Infanticide: An Anthropological Analysis, Infanticide and the Value of Life*. Buffalo, NY: Prometheus Books.
19. Birdsell, J. B. 1969. *Some Predictions*.
20. DeBurgh, W. G. 1924. *The Legacy of the Ancient World*. New York: Macmillan.
21. Eyben, M. 1980. *Family Planning in Greco-Roman Antiquity, Ancient Society*, 11/12: 5-82.

22. Becker, H. and R. Hill, eds, 1955. *Family, Marriages and Parenthood.* Boston: D. C. Heath Company.
23. Dickeman, M. 1975. *Demographic Consequences.*
24. Kennedy, R. 1972. *The Social Status of the Sexes and the Relative Mortality in Ireland, Readings and Population,* ed, W. Peterson. New York: Macmillan, 121-135.
25. Langer, W. L. 1974. *Infanticide: A Historical Survey, History of Childhood Quarterly,* 1(3): 353-365.
26. Pakrasi, K. 1970. *Female.*
27. Ryan, W. B. 1862. *Infanticide: Its Law, Prevalence, Prevention and History.* London, England: J. Churchill.
28. Sauer, R. 1978. *Infanticide and Abortion in 19th Century Britain, Population Studies,* 32: 81-93.
29. Sussman, G. D. 1975. *The Wet Nursing Business in 19th Century France, French Historical Studies,* 9: 304-328.
30. Sussman, G. D. 1977. *Parisian Infants and Wet Nurses in the Early 19th Century: A Statistical Study, Journal of Interdisciplinary History,* 7: 637-653.
31. Balikci, A. 1967. *Female.*
32. Williamson, L. 1971. *Infanticide.*
33. deMause, L. 1974. *The Evolution.*
34. Williamson, L. 1971. *Infanticide.*
35. Moll, A. 1913. *The Sexual Life of the Child.* New York: Macmillan Co.
36. Balikci, A. 1967. *Female.*
37. Cassidy, C. N. 1980. *Benign Neglect and Toddler Malnutrition, Social and Biological Predictors of Nutritional Status, Physical Growth and Neurological Development,* eds, Green and Johnson. New York: Academic Press, 101-131.
38. Dickeman, M. 1975. *Demographic Consequences.*
39. Eyben, M. 1980. *Family Planning.*
40. Langer, W. L. 1974. *Infanticide.*
41. McKee, L. 1982. *Preferential Care.*
42. Miller, B. D. 1981. *The Endangered Sex.* Ithaca, New York: Cornell University Press.
43. Hausfater, G. and S. D. Hrdy, eds. 1984. *Infanticide: Comparative and Evolutionary Perspectives.* New York: Aldine Publishing Co.

Chapter 2. Egypt: The Beginnings

A. The histories of Egypt comprise a library of their own. I have primarily used the following list as my resource in gathering

a general historical perspective, and balancing various view-
points. I discussed my views of this history with Dr.
Bierbrier and Dr. Feucht to make certain of the balance.

Aldred, C. 1965. *Egypt: To the End of the Old Kingdom.* New York:
McGraw-Hill.
Aldred, C. 1984. *The Egyptians.* London: Thames & Hudson.
Baines, J. and J. Melek 1958. *Atlas of Ancient Egypt, Facts of File Pub.* New
York.
Bianchi, R. S. 1980. *Museums of Egypt.* New York: *Newsweek.*
Bierbrier, M. 1982. *The Tomb-Builders of the Pharaohs.* New York: Charles
Scribners Sons.
Bronowski, J. 1973. *The Ascent of Man.* Boston: Little, Brown & Co.
Budge, E. A. W. 1967. *The Egyptian Book of the Dead.* New York: Dover
Press.
Coleca, A., D. Gioseffi, G. L. Mellini, and L. R. Collobi, 1967. *British
Museum,* London. New York: *Newsweek.*
Daniel, G., ed. 1977. *The Illustrated Encyclopedia of Archeology.* New York:
Thomas Y. Crowell Co.
Davis, V. L. 1978. *Ancient Egypt, National Geographic Service.* Wash-
ington.
de la Croix, H. and R. G. Tansey, ed. 1970. *Gardeners Art Through the
Ages.* New York: Harcourt, Brace & World, 30-114.
Donadoni, S. 1969. *The Egyptian Museum: Great Museums of the World.*
New York: *Newsweek.*
Durant, W. 1954. *Our Oriental Heritage, The Story of Civilization Part I.*
New York: Simon & Schuster.
Evans, H. 1979. *The Mystery of the Pyramids.* New York: Thomas Y.
Crowell.
Gardiner, A. 1961. *Egypt of the Pharaohs.* New York: Oxford University
Press.
Groenewegen-Frankfort, H. A. and B. Ashmole 1967. *The Library of Art
History: Vol. 1,* New York: New American Library, 7-111.
Grun, B. 1963. *Time Tables of History.* New York: Simon & Schuster.
Helck, W. and E. Otto 1972. *Lexikon der Agyptologie.* Wiesbaden: Har-
rassowitz, 423-439 (trans. by A. Marcotty).
International Graphics Society 1962. *The Arts of Mankind,* 6-34.
Langer, W. L. 1940. *An Encyclopedia of World History.* Boston: Houghton,
Mifflin, 1-36.
Myers, P. V. N. 1916. *Ancient History.* New York: Ginn & Co.
Peck, H. T. ed. 1965. *Harper's Dictionary of Classical Literature & Antiq-
uites.* New York: Cooper Square Pub.

Stierlien, H. 1978. *The World of the Pharaohs.* New York: Sunflower Books.

Tannahill, R. 1973. *Food in History.* New York: Stein & Day.

Van Sertima, I. ed. 1985. *Nile Valley Civilizations, Journal of African Civilizations,* Vol. 6.

Wells, H. G. 1940. *The Outline of History.* New York: Garden City Books.

1. Saadawi, N. E. L. 1981. *The Hidden Face of Eve: Women in the Arab World,* trans S. Hetata. Boston: Beacon Press.

2. Aldred, C. 1965. *Egypt: To the End of the Old Kingdom.* New York: McGraw-Hill.

3. Hallett, R. 1970. *Africa to 1875.* Ann Arbor: University of Michigan Press, 1-136.

4. Van Sertima, I. ed. 1985. *Nile Valley.*

5. Bierbrier, M. 1982. *The Tomb-Builders.*

6. Feucht, E. 1987. Agyptologisches Institut, University of Heidelberg (personal communication).

7. Baber, E. 1935. *Marriage and Family Life in Ancient Egypt, Social Forces,* 13: 409-414.

8. Bardis, P. D. 1966. *Selected Aspects of Family Life in Ancient Egypt, International Review of History and Political Science,* 3: 1-16.

9. Bardis, P. D. 1967. *Incest in Ancient Egypt, Indian Journal of Medicine,* 12(2): 12-40.

10. Erman, A. 1969. *Life in Ancient Egypt,* trans H. M. Tirard, New York: Benj. Blom Pub. (originally published 1894).

11. Montet, P. 1981. *Every Day Life In Egypt: In The Days of Rameses the Great,* trans. A. R. Maxwell-Hyslop and M. S. Drower, Philadelphia: University of Pennsylvania Press.

12. Seltman, C. 1956. *Women.*

13. Tannahill, R. 1973. *Food.*

14. Stierlien, H. 1978. *The World of the Pharaohs,* New York: Sunflower Books.

15. Trigger, B. G., B. J. Kemp, D. O'Connor, and A. B. Lloyd 1983. *Ancient Egypt: A Social History.* New York: Cambridge University Press.

16. Baber, E. 1935. *Marriage.*

17. Bardis, P. D. 1966, *Marriage and Family Customs in Ancient Egypt, Social Sciences,* 41: 229-245.

18. Feucht, E. 1986. *Researches in the Children and Family Life of Ancient Egypt* (Pre-Publication Draft) Heidelberg University (trans A. Marcotty).

19. Glanville, S. R. K. 1930. *Daily Life in Ancient Egypt: Introductions to Modern Knowledge*. London: Routledge and Sons, (16) 1-74.
20. Aldred, C. 1965. *Egypt*.
21. Bardis, P. D. 1966. *Selected Aspects*.
22. Bardis, P. D. 1966, *Marriage and Family Customs in Ancient Egypt, Social Sciences*, 41: 229-245.
23. Glanville, S. R. K. 1930. *Daily Life*.
24. Shorter, A. W. 1932. *Everyday Life in Ancient Egypt*. London: Sampson Low, Marston & Co.
25. Feucht, E. 1986. *Researches*.
26. Durant, W. 1954. *Our Oriental Heritage, The Story of Civilization Part I*. New York: Simon & Schuster.
27. Budge, E. A. W. 1967. *The Egyptian Book of the Dead*. New York: Dover Press.
28. Whitehead, C. 1968. *The Horus-Osiris Cycle: A Psychoanalytic Investigation, International Review of Psychoanalysis*, 13, I: 77-87.
29. Durant, W. 1954. *Our Oriental Heritage*.
30. Bianchi, R. S. 1980. *Museums*.
31. Coleca, A., et al. 1967. *British Museum*.
32. Daniel, G. ed. 1977. *The Illustrated Encyclopedia of Archeology*. New York: Thomas Y. Crowell.
33. Donadoni, S. 1969. *The Egyptian Museum*.
34. Groenewegen-Frankfort, H. A. and B. Ashmole 1967. *The Library of Art History: Vol. 1*. New York: New American Library, 7-111.
35. International Graphics Society, 1962. *The Arts*.
36. Bianchi, R. S. 1980. *Museums of Egypt*.
37. Coleca, A., et al. 1967. *British Museum*.
38. Daniel, G. ed. 1977. *The Illustrated Encyclopedia*.
39. Donadoni, S. 1969. *The Egyptian Museum*.
40. Groenewegen-Frankfort, H. A. and B. Ashmole 1967. *The Library*.
41. International Graphics Society, 1962. *The Arts of Mankind*, 6-34.
42. Baber, R. E. 1935. *Marriage*.
43. Bardis, P. D. 1966. *Selected Aspects*.
44. Bardis, P. D. 1966, *Marriage*.
45. Durant, W. 1954. *Our Oriental Heritage*.
46. Erman, A. 1969. *Life in Ancient Egypt*.
47. Feucht, E. 1986. *Researches*.
48. Glanville, S. R. K. 1930. *Daily Life*.
49. Van Sertima, I. ed. 1985. *Nile*.
50. Mailer, N. 1983. *Ancient Evenings*. Boston: Little Brown & Co.
51. Scott, N. E. 1967. *The Home Life of the Ancient Egyptians*. New York: Metropolitan Museum of Art.

52. Bardis, P. D. 1966, *Marriage.*
53. Erman, A. 1969. *Life.*
54. Feucht, E. 1986. *Researches.*
55. Glanville, S. R. K. 1930. *Daily Life.*
56. Montet, P. 1981. *Everyday Life.*
57. Scott, N. E. 1967. *The Home Life.*
58. Shorter, A. W. 1932. *Everyday Life.*
59. Trigger, B. G., *et al.* 1983. *Ancient Egypt.*
60. Budge, E. A. W. 1967. *The Egyptian.*
61. Durant, W. 1954. *Our Oriental Heritage.*
62. Whitehead, C. 1968. *The Horus-Osiris Cycle.*
63. Baber, R. E. 1935. *Marriage.*
64. Bardis, P. D. 1966. *Marriage.*
65. Bardis, P. D. 1967. *Incest.*
66. Bixler, R. H. 1983. *Sibling Incest in the Royal Families of Egypt, Peru, and Hawaii, The Journal of Sex Research,* 18:(3) 264-281.
67. Middleton, R. 1962. *Brother-Sister and Father-Daughter Marriage in Ancient Egypt, American Sociologic Review,* 27,5: 603-610.
68. Pomeroy, S. B. 1975. *Goddesses, Whores, Wives and Slaves.* New York: Schocken Books, 1-16.
69. Seltman, C. 1956. *Women.*
70. Trigger, B. G., et al. 1983. *Ancient Egypt.*
71. Aldred, C. 1965. *Egypt.*
72. Aldred, C. 1984. *The Egyptians.*
73. Durant, W. 1954. *Our Oriental Heritage.*
74. Gardiner, A. 1961. *Egypt.*
75. Stierlien, H. 1978. *The World.*
76. Durant, W. 1954. *Our Oriental Heritage.*
77. Bardis, P. D. 1967. *Incest.*
78. Bixler, R. H. 1983. *Sibling Incest.*
79. Durant, W. 1954. *Our Oriental Heritage.*
80. Mailer, N. 1983. *Ancient.*
81. Middleton, R. 1962. *Brother-Sister.*
82. Mailer, N. 1983. *Ancient.*
83. Feucht, E. 1986. *Researches.*
84. Budge, E. A. W. 1967. *The Egyptian.*
85. Davis, V. L. 1978. *Ancient.*
86. Durant, W. 1954. *Our Oriental Heritage.*
87. Myers, P. V. N. 1916. *Ancient History.*
88. Wells, H. G. 1940. *The Outline.*
89. Whitehead, C. 1968. *The Horus-Osiris Cycle.*

90. Aldred, C. 1965. *Egypt.*
91. Aldred, C. 1984. *The Egyptians.*
92. Brierbrier, M. 1982. *The Tomb-Builders.*
93. Bronowski, J. 1973. *The Ascent.*
94. Davis, V. L. 1978. *Ancient.*
95. Durant, W. 1954. *Our Oriental Heritage.*
96. Shorter, A. W. 1932. *Everyday Life.*
97. Trigger, B. G., et al. 1983. *Ancient Egypt.*
98. Gardiner, A. 1961. *Egypt.*
99. Montet, P. 1981. *Everyday Life.*
100. Baber, R. E. 1935. *Marriage.*
101. Bardis, P. D. 1966, *Selected Aspects.*
102. Feucht, E. 1986. *Researches.*
103. Middleton, R. 1962. *Brother-Sister.*
104. Montet, P. 1981. *Everyday Life.*
105. Pomeroy, S. B. 1975. *Goddesses.*
106. Scott, N. E. 1967. *The Home Life.*
107. Seltman, C. 1956. *Women.*
108. Aldred, C. 1984. *The Egyptians.*
109. Baber, R. E. 1935. *Marriage.*
110. Bardis, P. D. 1966. *Selected Aspects.*
111. Bardis, P. D. 1966. *Marriage.*
112. Durant, W. 1954. *Our Oriental Heritage.*
113. Erman, A. 1969. *Life.*
114. Glanville, S. R. K. 1930. *Daily Life.*
115. Montet, P. 1981. *Everyday Life.*
116. Pomeroy, S. B. 1975. *Goddesses.*
117. Seltman, C. 1956. *Women.*
118. Bardis, P. D. 1967. *Contraception In Ancient Egypt, Indian Journal of the History,* 12(2): 1-3.
119. Shorter, A. W. 1932. *Everyday Life.*

Chapter 3. Greece: The Heights and the Depths

A. To gain perspective on Greek history and its complicated interweaving with the cultures of various ethnic groups over an extended period I utilized the material on this list, and of course the historical material in the bibliography of the other

Mediterranean cultures I have written about in this book. You will find the books by Bonnard, Durant, and Tuchman fascinating and enlightening.

Bonnard, A. 1959. *Greek Civilization*. New York: Macmillan.
Durant, W. 1966. *The Life of Greece*. New York: Simon & Schuster.
Durant, W. 1954. *Our Oriental Heritage*.
Grun, B. 1979. *The Timetables of History*. New York: Simon & Schuster.
Kitto, H. D. F. 1951. *The Greeks*. Middlesex: Penguin Press.
Moll, A. 1913. *Ancient Society*. New York: Meridian Press.
Robinson, C. E. 1948. *Hellas*. New York: Pantheon Books.
Tannahill, R. 1973. *Food in History*. New York: Stein & Day.
Thompson, G. 1949. *Studies in Ancient Greek Society I: The Prehistoric Aegean*. New York: International Press.
Tuchman, B. W. 1984. *The March of Folly*. New York: Knopf.

1. Becker, H. and R. Hill, eds. 1955. *Family Marriage and Parenthood*. Boston: D. C. Heath.
2. Bonnard, A. 1959. *Greek Civilization*. New York: Macmillan Co.
3. Durant, W. 1966. *The Life*.
4. Durant, W. 1966. *Our Oriental Heritage*.
5. Ehrenberg, V. 1943. *The People of Aristophanes*. Oxford: Blackwell.
6. Flaceliere, R. 1964. *Daily Life in Greece At The Time of Pericles*. New York: Macmillan.
7. Harrison, A. R. W. 1968. *The Law of Athens: The Family and Property*. Oxford: Clarendon Press.
8. Kitto, H. D. F. 1951. *The Greeks*.
9. Lacey, W. K. 1968. *The Family in Classical Greece*. Ithaca: Cornell University Press.
10. Moll, A. 1913. *Ancient Society*.
11. Robinson, C. E. 1948. *Hellas*. New York: Pantheon Books.
12. Slater, P. E. 1968. *The Glory of Hera: Greek Mythology and The Greek Family*. Boston: Beacon Press.
13. Thompson, G. D. 1949. *Studies*.
14. Wolf, H. J. 1944. *Marriage Law and Family Organization in Ancient Athens, Tradition*, 2: 43-95.
15. deBeauvoir, S. 1953. *The Second Sex*. New York: Knopf.
16. Ireland, N. O. 1970. *Index to Women of the World from Ancient to Modern Times: Biographies and Portraits*. Mass.: Faxon.
17. Levy, O. 1964. *The Greek Woman*. New York: Russell Press.

18. Light, H. 1934. *Sexual Life in Ancient Greece*. New York: American Anthropological Society.
19. Pomeroy, S. B. 1973. Selected Bibliography on Women in Antiquity, *Arethusa*. Westwood, Mass.: F. W. Faxon Co. 6 (1) 125-157.
20. Seltman, C. 1956. *Women*.
21. Tannahill, R. 1980. *Sex*.
22. Wolf, H. J. 1944. *Marriage Law*.
23. Dingwall, E. J. 1925. *Male Infibulation*. London: J. Beale & Sons—Danielsson Ltd.
24. Hertz, J. H. ed. 1981. *Pentateuch Haftorahs*. London: Soncino Press.
25. Kaplan, K. J., M. W. Schwartz, and M. M. Kaplan, 1984. *The Family: Biblical and Psychological Foundations, Journal of Psychology and Judaism*. 8(2) 132pp.
26. Thompson, G. D. 1949. *Studies*.
27. Flaceliere, R. 1964. *Daily Life*.
28. deMause, L. ed. *History*.
29. Ende, A. 1983. Children in History, *Journal of Psychohistory*. 11(1).
30. Garrison, F. H. 1965. Abt-Garrison History of Pediatrics, *Pediatrics*. Philadelphia: Saunders Co., Vol. 1.
31. Payne, G. H. 1916. *The Child and Human Progress*. New York: G. P. Putnam.
32. Pieper, A. 1966. *Chronik Kinderheilkunde*. Leipzig: Veb Georg Thiem.
33. Ruhrah, J. 1925. *Pediatrics of the Past*. New York: P. B. Hoeber.
34. Devereux, G. 1967. *Greek Pseudo-Homosexuality and the Greek Miracle, Symbolae Osloenses*. 42: 69-92.
35. Durant, W. 1966. *The Life*.
36. Light, H. 1934. *Sexual Life*.
37. Marmor, J., ed. 1980. *Homosexual Behavior*. New York: Basic Books.
38. Shiner, L. E. 1980. *The Darker Side of Hellas: Sexuality and Violence in Ancient Greece, Psychohistory Review*. 9(1) 111-135.
39. Hertz, J. H. ed. 1981. *Pentateuch*.
40. Manheim, R. 1967. *Myth, Religion and Mother Rites: Selected Writings of J. J. Bachofen*. Princeton, NJ: Princeton University Press, Bollingen Series 85.
41. Trexler, R. 1973. *Infanticide in Florence: New Sources and First Results*. New York: A History of Childhood Quarterly, 1: 98-116.
42. deMause, L. ed. *History of Childhood*, New York: Psychohistory Press.
43. Ende, A. 1983. *Children*.
44. Hertz, J. H., ed. 1981. *Pentateuch*.
45. Ryan, W. B. 1862. *Infanticide*.

46. Shiner, L. E. 1980. *The Darker Side*.
47. Trexler, R. 1973. *Infanticide*.
48. Williamson, L. 1971. *Infanticide: An Anthropological Analysis, Infanticide and the Value of Life*. Buffalo: Prometheus Books.
49. Durant, W. 1966. *The Life*.
50. Flaceliere, R. 1964. *Daily Life*.
51. Harrison, A. R. W. 1968. *The Law*.
52. Shiner, L. E. 1980. *The Darker Side*.
53. Tuchman, B. W. 1984. *The March*.
54. Tannahill, R. 1973. *Food*.
55. Durant, W. 1966. *The Life*.
56. Manheim, R. 1967. *Myth*.
57. Slater, P. E. 1968. *The Glory of Hera: Greek Mythology and The Greek Family*. Boston: Beacon Press.

Chapter 4. The Hebrews: And God Spoke to the People

A. The history of the Hebrews is intimately tied to that of the Egyptians, Greeks, and Romans; yet they had their own logical development. Their history particularly is inextricably tied to their religion. To help the reader in following this complicated story I have given an overview of their history utilizing the texts listed. I would like to draw your attention to the following authors on this list: ben-Sasson, Durant, and Sacher, as particularly helpful in giving more information. I personally enjoyed books not on this list—Howard Fast's *The History of the Jews*, and Max Dimot's *Jews, God and History*.

ben-Sasson, B. H. 1976. *The History of the Jewish People*. Mass: Harvard University.
Comay, J. 1974. *Who's Who in Jewish History*. New York: David MacKay Co.
Comay, J. 1981. *The Diaspora Story*. Jerusalem: Steimatzky Agency.
deVauz, R. 1961. *The Old Testament, Its Life Institutions*. New York: McGraw-Hill.
Durant, W. 1954. *The Story of Civilization: Part I Our Oriental Heritage*. New York: Simon & Schuster.

Epstein, T. 1959. *Judaism A Historical Presentation*. Baltimore: Penguin Books.

Fackenhein, E. L. 1970. *God's Presence in History: Jewish Affirmations and Philosophical Reflections*. New York: Harper & Row.

Hertz, J. H., ed. 1981. *The Pentateuch Haftorahs*. London: Soncino Press.

Buttrick, G. A. 1962. *Interpreter's Dictionary of the Bible*. New York: Abingdon Press.

Kaniel, M. 1979. *Judaism*. Dorsett, England: Blanford Press.

Kenyon, K. N. 1974. *Digging Up Jerusalem*. London: Ernest Benn.

Rabinowitz, L. I., ed. 1973. *Encyclopaedia Judaica*. Jerusalem: Keter Publishing Ltd.

Landay, J. M. 1971. *Silent Cities, Sacred Stones*. New York: McCall Books.

Parrinder, G., ed. 1971. *World Religions from Ancient History to the Present*. New York: Facts On File Publications.

Pearlman, M. 1980. *Digging Up the Bible*. New York: William Morrow & Co.

Sacher, H. M. 1970. *A History of Israel*. New York: Alfred A. Knopf.

Werblowsky, R., J. Zwi, and G. Wigoder, ed. 1965. *The Encyclopedia of the Jewish Religion*, New York: Holt Rinehart Winston.

B. The Hebrews were a God-intoxicated people who wrote extensively on their religion; more than any other peoples in the history of the world. To summarize this religion is on one hand simple (see Hillel) and too complex except for a lifetime student (e.g., the Kabbalah, Talmud). The following list I utilized to obtain understanding and a broader view. Of course, I was most interested in how the religion directly applies to the family. The following authors are particularly recommended: Arieti, Hertz, and Soares.

Arieti, S. 1981. *Abraham and the Contemporary Mind*. New York: Basic Books.

Arlow, J. A. 1951. *The Consecration of the Prophet*. Psychoanalytic Quarterly, 20: 374-397.

Boker, B. Z. 1981. *The Jewish Mystical Tradition*. New York: Pilgrim Press. York,

Epstein, T. 1959. *Judaism A Historical Presentation*. Baltimore: Penguin Books.

Fackenhein, E. L. 1970. *God's Presence In History: Jewish Affirmations and Philosophical Reflections*. New York: Harper & Row.

Ganfried, S. 1927. *Code of Jewish Law* (*Kitzur Schulchan Aruch*). New York: Hebrew Publishing Co.

Gaster, T. H. 1980. *The Holy and the Profane*. New York: William Morrow.

Hertz, J. H., ed. 1981. *The Pentateuch*.

Kaniel, M. 1979. *Judaism*.

Klagsbrun, F. 1980. *Voices of Wisdom: Jewish Ideals and Ethics for Everyday Living*. New York: Pantheon Books.

MacGregor, S. L. and S. W. Mathers 1968. *The Kabbalah Unveiled*. New York: Beech Main Pub.

Parrinder, G. ed. 1971. *World Religions*.

Soares, T. J. 1915. *The Social Institutions and Ideas of the Bible*. New York: Abingdon Press.

Trachtenberg, J. 1939. *Jewish Magic and Superstition*. New York: Behrman Jewish Book House.

Werblowsky, R., J. Zwi, and G. Wigoder, eds. *The Encyclopedia*.

1. Durant, W. 1954. *Our Oriental Heritage*.
2. Sacher, H. M. 1979. *A History of Israel*. New York: Alfred A. Knopf.
3. Hertz, J. H. ed. 1981. *The Pentateuch*.
4. Bardis, P. D. 1963. Main Features of the Ancient Hebrew Family, *Social Science*, 38, 168–193.
5. Ellis, A. B. 1983. Marriage and Kinship among the Ancient Israelites, *Popular Science Monthly*, 42, 325-337.
6. Kaplan, K. J., M. W. Schwartz, and M. M. Kaplan 1984. The Family: Biblical and Psychological Foundations. *Journal of Psychology and Judaism*, 8, 2.
7. Mendelsohn, I. 1948. The Family in the Ancient Near East. *Biblical Archeologist*, 11: 24-40.
8. Neufield, E. 1944. *Ancient Hebrew Marriage Laws*. New York: Longmans, Green & Co.
9. Patai, R. 1959. *Sex and Family in the Bible in the Middle East*. New York: Doubleday & Co.
10. Soares, T. J. 1915. *The Social Institutions*.
11. Avidor-Hacohen, S. *The Child in the Bible*. Tel Aviv: World WIZO Dept. of Education.
12. Bardis, P. D. 1963. Main Feature of the Ancient Hebrew Family. *Social Science*, 38: 168-193.
13. deVauz, R. 1961. *The Old Testament*.
14. Feldman, N. 1918. *The Jewish Child in History, Folklore, Biology and Sociology*. New York: Bloch Publishing Co.

15. Gerard, J. H. 1976. *Children and the Aggada*. New York: Hebrew William College, Jewish Institute of Religion.
16. Koltun, L. ed. 1973. *The Jewish Woman*. Waltham, Mass: Response Publisher.
17. Miner, P. 1948. *The Status of the Minor in Tannaitic Literature: Legal, Social and Ethical Aspects*. Cincinnati: Hebrew Union College.
18. Babylonian Talmud (translation). Cincinnati: Hebrew Union College.
19. Finesilver, A. 1980. *The Talmud for Today*. New York: St. Martins Press.
20. Jerusalem Talmud (translation). Cincinnati: Union College.
21. Steinsaltz, A. 1976. *The Essential Talmud*. London: Weidenfeld and Nikolsen.
22. Bardis, P. D. 1963. *Main Feature*.
23. Ellis, A. B. 1983. *Marriage*.
24. Neufield, E. 1944. *Ancient Hebrew*.
25. Avidor-Hacohen, S. *The Child*.
26. Feldman, N. 1918. *The Jewish Child*.
27. Gerard, J. H. 1976. *Children*.
28. Kaplan, K. J., et al. 1984. *The Family*.
29. Miner, P. 1948. *The Status*.
30. Ganfried, S. 1927. *Code of Jewish Law* (*Kitzur Schulchan Aruch*). New York: Hebrew Publishing Co.
31. Miner, P. 1948. *The Status*.
32. Buttrick, G. A. 1962. *Interpreter's Dictionary*.
33. Koltun, L., ed. 1973. *The Jewish Woman*.
34. Patai, R. 1959. *Sex and Family*.
35. Koltun, L. ed. 1973. *The Jewish Woman*.
36. Petai, R. 1959. *Sex and Family*.
37. Ganfried, S. 1927. *Code*.
38. Comay, J. 1981. *The Diaspora*.
39. Finesilver, A. 1980. *The Talmud*.
40. Klagsbrun, F. 1980. *Voices of Wisdom: Jewish Ideals and Ethics for Everyday Living*. New York: Pantheon Books.
41. Montefiore, C. G. and H. Loewe. 1974. *A Rabbinic Anthology*. New York: Schocken Books.
42. Werblowsky, R. et al. 1965. *The Encyclopedia*.
43. *Interpreter's Dictionary*. 1962.
44. ben-Sasson, B. H. 1976. *The History*.
45. Comay, J. 1981. *The Diaspora*.
46. Durant, W. 1954. *Our Oriental Heritage*.
47. Sacher, H. M. 1979. *A History*.

48. Babylonian Talmud.
49. Jerusalem Talmud.
50. Finesilver, A. 1980. *The Talmud.*
51. Hertz, J. H., ed. 1981. *The Pentateuch.*
52. Miner, P. 1948. *The Status.*
53. Montefiore, C. G., and H. Loewe. 1976. *A Rabbinic Anthology.*
54. Soares, T. J. 1915. *The Social Institutions.*
55. Steinsaltz, A. 1976. *The Essential Talmud.*
56. Fackenhein, E. L. 1970. *God's Presence.*
57. Finesilver, A. 1980. *The Talmud.*
58. Montefiore, C. G., and H. Loewe. 1974. *A Rabbinic Anthology.*
59. Steinsaltz, A. 1976. *The Essential Talmud.*
60. Durant, W. 1954. *Our Oriental Heritage.*
61. Hertz, J. H. ed. 1981. *The Pentateuch.*
62. Patai, R. 1959. *Sex and Family.*

Chapter 5. Rome: The Power and Some Glory

A. The history of the Roman Empire has a certain familiarity. Yet this very familiarity has prevented seeing this culture in the general flow of history, as well as its functioning on the less dramatic stage of the family. I have utilized the following list of books (along with other texts on the other chapters) to get this broader perspective, primarily of the human side of Rome. Two authors' books are outstanding: Durant and Gibbon. I cannot praise the brilliant work by Gibbon enough. Any page opened at random among the many volumes of this work can be read with delight and fresh insight.

Durant, W. 1944. *Caesar and Christ—The Story of Civilization, Part III,* New York: Simon & Schuster.
Fustel, D. D. and N. Denis, 1980. *The Ancient City.* Baltimore: Johns Hopkins University Press.
Gibbon, E. 1946. *The Decline and Fall of the Roman Empire.* New York: The Heritage Press (originally published 1781).
Grun, B. 1963. *The Time Tables of History.* New York: Simon & Schuster.
Suetonius. 1965. *The Lives of the Twelve Caesars,* trans. O. Holland. New York: Heritage Press.

Tannahill, R. 1973. *Food*.
Hamilton, E. 1932. *The Roman Way*. New York: W. W. Norton & Co.

1. Aerahamfe, D. 1979. Images of Childhood in Early Byzantine, New York: *Journal of Psychohistory*. 6:(4) 497-517.
2. Luck, G. 1985. *Arcana Mundi*. Baltimore: Johns Hopkins University Press.
3. Pomeroy, S. B. 1975. *Goddesses*.
4. Hertz, J. H. ed. 1981. *The Pentateuch*.
5. Becker, H. and R. Hall ed. 1955. *Family, Marriage and Parenthood*. Boston: D. C. Heath Co.
6. Durant, W. 1944. *Caesar*.
7. Gibbon, E. 1946. *The Decline*.
8. Johnston, H. W. 1903. *The Private Life of the Romans*. 1903. Scott Foresman & Co.
9. Becker, H. and R. Hall, ed. 1955. *Family*.
10. Durant, W. 1944. *Caesar*.
11. Ende, A. 1983. *Children*.
12. Fine, R. 1985. *The Meaning of Love and Human Experience*. New York: John Wiley & Sons.
13. Garrison, F. H. and Abt-Garrison. 1965. *History of Pediatrics, Pediatrics Vol. 1*. Philadelphia: Saunders Company.
14. Gibbon, E. 1946. *The Decline*.
15. Lefkowitz, M. R. and M. B. Fant. 1982. *Women's Life in Greece and Rome*. Baltimore: The Johns Hopkins University Press.
16. Payne, G. H. 1916. *The Child and Human Progress*. New York: G. P. Putnam & Son.
17. Ruhrah, J. 1925. *Pediatrics of the Past*. New York: P. B. Hoeber.
18. Seltman, C. 1956. *Women in Antiquity*.
19. Becker, H. and R. Hall, ed. 1955. *Family*.
20. Gibbon, E. 1946. *The Decline*.
21. Johnston, H. W. 1903. *The Private Life*.
22. Ibid.
23. Lefkowitz, M. R. and M. B. Fant. 1982. *Women's Life*.
24. Pomeroy, S. B. 1975. *Goddesses*.
25. Trexler, *Infanticide*.
26. Suetonius, 1965. *The Lives*.
27. Becker, H. and R. Hall, ed. 1955. *Family*.
28. deMause, L., ed. 1974. *The History*.
29. Ende, A., 1983. *Children*.

30. Garrison, F. H. and Abt-Garrison, 1965. History.
31. Payne, G. H. 1916. *The Child.*
32. Ruhrah, J. 1925. *Pediatrics.*
33. Ryan, W. B. 1862. *Infanticide.*
34. Trexler, *Infanticide* (after deMause—History of Childhood).
35. Williamson, L. 1971. *Infanticide.*
36. deMause, L., ed. 1974. *The History.*
37. Pieper, A. 1951. *Chronik.*
38. Fustel, D. D. and N. Denis. 1980. *The Ancient City.*
39. Gibbon, E. 1946. *The Decline.*
40. Johnston, H. W. 1903. *The Private Life.*
41. Lefkowitz, M. R. and M. B. Fant. 1982. *Women's Life.*
42. Petronius, 1965. *The Satyricon and the Fragments*, Baltimore: Penguin Press.
43. Pomeroy, S. B. 1975. *Goddesses.*
44. Suetonius. 1965. *The Lives.*
45. Ibid.
46. deMause, L. ed. 1974. *The History.*
47. Suetonius. 1965. *The Lives.*
48. Ibid.
49. Ibid.
50. Ibid.
51. Hertz, J. H. ed. 1981. *The Pentateuch.*
52. Tannahill, R. 1973. *Food.*
53. Ibid.
54. Suetonius, 1965. *The Lives.*
55. Aerahamfe, D. 1979. *Images of Childhood.*
56. Gibbon, E. 1946. *The Decline.*
57. Edwards, W. D., W. J. Gabel, and F. E. Hosmer. 1986. On the Physical Death of Jesus Christ. *Journal of the American Medical Association.* 255:(11) 1455-1463.
58. Suetonius. 1965. *The Lives.*
59. Ibid.
60. Gibbon, E. 1946. *The Decline.*

Chapter 6. China: East Meets West

A. The history of China is not only extensive, it also has been distorted at times by Western writers. I have utilized the following list along with consultations with Chinese experts (both native Chinese and Occidental) to obtain a more accurate perspective. In addition to Durant's brilliant overview, I would like to recommend four other books on this list that helped enormously in my understanding of the long and magnificent history of China: Ebrey, Ho, Li, and Ronan.

Chan, Wing'tsit. 1963. *A Source Book in Chinese Philosophy*. Princeton, N.J.: Princeton University Press, 1963.

Chang, C., ed. 1975. *The Making of China*. Englewood Cliffs, N.J.: Prentice Hall.

Chang, Kwang-chih. 1980. *Shang Civilization*. New Haven, Conn.: Yale University Press, 88, 119, 121.

Confucius. *The Hsia King* (classic of Filial Piety).

Creel, H. G. 1937. *The Birth of China*. New York: Frederick Ungar.

Creel, H. G. 1970. *The Origins of Statecraft in China*, Chicago, Ill.: The University of Chicago Press, Vol. 1.

deBarry, W. T., W. Chang, and B. Watson. 1960. *Sources of Chinese Tradition*. New York: Columbia University Press, Vol. 1.

Durant, W. 1954. *The Story*.

Ebrey, P. B. 1981. *Chinese Civilization and Society*. New York: The Free Press.

Elvin, N. 1973. *The Pattern of the Chinese Past*. Stanford, Calif.: Stanford University Press.

Hao, Q., H. Chen, and S. Ru. *Out of China's Earth: Archaeology Discoveries in the Peoples Republic of China*, New York: Henry N. Abrams.

Ho, P. 1975. *The Cradle of the East*, Hong Kong: The Chinese University of Hong Kong and Chicago, Ill: University of Chicago Press.

Hucker, C. O. 1975. *China's Imperial Past*. Stanford, Calif.: Stanford University Press.

Lach, D. F. 1965. *Asia in the Making of Europe*. Chicago, Ill.: University of Chicago Press, Vol. 1.

Li, D. J. 1971. *The Ageless Chinese*. New York: Charles Scribners Sons.

Maspero, H. 1978. *China in Antiquity*. Amherst: University of Massachusetts Press.

Rawson, J. 1980. *Ancient China's Art and Archaeology*. New York: Harper & Row.

Ronan, C. A. 1978. *The Shorter Science and Civilization in China*. New York: Cambridge University Press.

Tannahil, R. 1973. *Food*.

Woo, K. D. 1982. *The Chinese Heritage*. New York: Crown Publishers.

Weiner, P. P. ed. 1968. *Dictionary of the History of Ideas*. New York: Charles Scribner's Sons.

Wong, L. 1932. *History of Chinese Medicine*. Tientsin, China: Tientsin Press.

B. The Chinese family has been looked at superficially and often with distortions. To obtain fuller understanding without obfuscating biases has been my object. I was helped extensively by reading many texts including the following. Of particular value I want to recommend Hsu's book, *Under the Ancestor's Shadow*.

Buxbaum, D. C. 1978. *Chinese Family Law and Social Change*. Seattle, Wash.: University of Washington Press.

Confucius. The Hsia King.

deBarry, W. T., W. Chang, and B. Watson 1960. *Sources of Chinese Tradition*. New York: Columbia University Press. Vol. 1.

Ebrey, P. B. 1981. *Chinese Civilization*.

Fei, H. T. 1939. *Peasant Life in China*. London: Routledge.

Freedman, M. 1970. *Family and Kinship in Chinese Society*. Stanford, Calif.: Stanford University Press.

Gernet, J. 1962. *Daily Life in China on the Eve of the Mongol Invasion*. New York: Macmillan Co. 1250-1276.

Hsu, F. L. K. 1967. *Under the Ancestor's Shadow*. Stanford, Calif: Stanford University Press.

Lang, O. 1946. *Chinese Family and Society*. New Haven, Conn.: Yale University Press.

Liu, H. W. 1959. *The Traditional Chinese Clan Rites*, Association for Asian Studies. New York: J. J. Augustin.

Loewe, M. 1968. *Everyday Life in Early Imperial China*. New York: Harper & Row.

Rubin, V. A., trans. S. I. Levine, 1976. *Individual and State in Ancient China*. New York: Columbia University Press.

Wilkinson, H. P. 1926. *The Family in Classical China*. Shanghai, China: Kelly & Walsh Publisher.

Yah King. *The Book of Changes*, from 34th Century B.C. to 12th Century B.C.

Yih'fu, R. 1961. *Changing Structure of the Chinese Family.*, Bulletin Dept. of Archaeology and Anthropology, Taiwan University, 1-14.

1. Ronan, C. A. 1978. *The Shorter Science*.
2. Veith, I. 1972. *The Yellow Emperor's Classic of Internal Medicine* (Hujan Ti Nei Ching Su Wen). Berkeley, Calif.: University of California Press.
3. Ware, J. R. 1966. *Alchemy, Medicine and Religion in the China of A.D. 320* (Nei Pien of Ku Hung). Cambridge, Mass.: MIT Press.
4. Wong, L. 1932. *History*.
5. Durant, W. 1954. *The Story*. p. 735.
6. Chan, Wing'tsit, 1963. *A Source Book*.
7. deBarry, W. T., W. Chang, and B. Watson. 1960. *Sources*.
8. Liu, H. W. 1959. *The Traditional*.
9. Chan, Wing'tsit. 1963. *A Source*.
10. Durant, W. 1954. *The Story*.
11. Woo, K. D. 1982. *The Chinese*.
12. Weiner, P. P. ed. 1968. *Dictionary of the History of Ideas*. New York: Charles Scribner's Sons.
13. Lee, B. J. 1981. *Female Infanticide in China, Historical Reflections*. 8:163-177.
14. Schaefer, E. A. *Ritual Exposure In Ancient China*. Berkeley, Calif.: University of California Press.
15. Chang, Kwang-chih. 1980. *Shang Civilization*. New Haven, Conn.: Yale University Press, 88, 119, 121.
16. Schaefer, E. A. *Ritual*.
17. *Science News*. August 1984. 126: 89.
18. *Spring and Autumn Annals from the State of Lu*. 722-481 B.C.
19. Buxbaum, D. C. 1978. *Chinese Family*.
20. Confucius. The Hsia King.
21. deBarry, W. T., W. Chang, and B. Watson. 1960. *Sources*.
22. Durant, W. 1954. *The Story*.
23. Ebrey, P. B. 1981. *Chinese*.
24. Fei, H. T. 1939. *Peasant Life in China*. London: Routledge.
25. Freedman, M. 1970. *Family*.
26. Hsu, F. L. K. 1967. *Under*.
27. Lang, O. 1946. *Chinese*.
28. Confucius, The Hsia King.
29. Freedman, M. 1970. *Family*.
30. Hsu, F. L. K. 1967. *Under*.
31. Fei, H. T. 1939. *Peasant*.
32. Fine, R. 1985. *The Meaning of Love and Human Experience*. New York: John Wiley and Sons.
33. Freedman, M. 1970. *Family*.

34. *Spring and Autumn Annals.*
35. Creel, H. G. 1970. *The Origins.*
36. Ebrey, P. B. 1981. *Chinese.*
37. Ku, P. 1974. *Courtier and Commoner in Ancient China*: from the History of the Former Han; trans. B. Watson. New York: Columbia University Press.
38. Rubin, V. A. 1976. trans. S. I. Levine, 1976. *Individual and State in Ancient China.* New York: Columbia University Press.
39. Bodde, D. and C. Morris. 1967. *Law in Imperial China.* Cambridge, Mass: Harvard University Press.
40. Buxbaum, D. C. 1978. *Chinese.*
41. Ch'u, T'ung-tsu. 1915. *Law In Society In Traditional China.* Paris: Mouton & Co.
42. Staunton, G. T., trans. 1966. *Ta Tsing Leu Lee (Fundamental Laws of the Penal Code of China)*, originally published 1810. Taiwan: Ch'eng-wen Publishing Co.
43. Bodde, D. and C. Morris 1967. *Law.*
44. Ibid.
45. Staunton, G. T. 1966. *Ta Tsing Leu Lee.*
46. Beurdeley, M. 1969. *Chinese Erotic Art.* Vermont: Charles E. Tuttle Co.
47. Fei, H. T. 1939. *Peasant.*
48. Fine, R. 1985. *The Meaning.*
49. Freedman, M. 1970. *Family.*
50. Needham, J. 1954. *Science and Civilization in China: Sexual Techniques.* Cambridge, England: Cambridge University Press, Vol. 2.
51. Ronan, C. A. 1978. *The Shorter Science.*
52. *Spring and Autumn Annals.*
53. Chang, Kwang-chih. 1980. *Shang.*
54. Creel, H. G. 1937. *The Birth.*
55. Maspero, H. 1978. *China.*
56. Rawson, J. 1980. *Ancient.*
57. Needham, J. 1954. *Science.*
58. van Gulik, R. H. 1974. *Sexual Life In Ancient China.* Leiden: E. J. Brill Publishing.
59. Ware, J. R. 1966. *Alchemy.*
60. van Gulik, R. H. 1974. *Sexual Life.*
61. Beurdeley, M. 1969. *Chinese.*
62. Ibid.
63. Hucker, C. O. 1961. *The Traditional Chinese State in Ming Times.* Tucson, Arizona: University of Arizona Press.

64. Ibid.
65. Levy, H. S. 1966. *Chinese Footbinding*. New York: W. Rawls.
66. Needham, J. 1954. *Science*.
67. van Gulik, R. H. 1974. *Sexual Life*.
68. Chang, Kwang-chih. 1980. *Shang*.
69. Ku, P. 1974. *Courtier*.
70. Chang, C., ed. 1975. *The Making*.
71. Durant, W. 1954. *The Story*.
72. Elvin, N. 1973. *The Pattern*.
73. Gernet, J. 1962. *Daily Life*.
74. Hucker, C. O. 1961. *The Traditional*.
75. Maspero, H. 1978. *China*.
76. Ronan, C. A. 1978. *The Shorter Science*.
77. Schurmann, F. and O. Schell, eds. *The China Reader: Imperial China: The Decline of the Last Dynasty and the Origins of Modern China*. New York: Random House.
78. Breiner, S. J. 1985. *Child Abuse Patterns: Comparison of Ancient Western Civilization and Traditional China, Analytic Psychotherapy & Psychopathology*, 2:1 27-50.
79. Breiner, S. J. 1980. *Early Childhood*.
80. Hsu, F. L. K. 1967. *Under*.
81. Lee, B. J. 1981. *Female*.
82. Wilkinson, H. P. 1926. *The Family*.
83. Yih'fu, R. 1961. *Changing Structure*.
84. Breiner, M. S. 1979. *Economic Change in Late Imperial China*. Master's thesis. Ann Arbor: University of Michigan.
85. Breiner, S. J. 1985. *Child Abuse*.
86. Breiner, S. J. 1980. *Early Childhood*.
87. Gernet, J. 1962. *Daily Life*.
88. Marsden, W. 1948. trans. & ed. 1948. *The Travels of Marco Polo the Venetian*, New York: International Collectors Library.
89. Hucker, C. O. 1961. *The Traditional*.
90. Schurmann, F. and O. Schell, eds. 1961. *The China Reader*.
91. Ho, D. Y. E. 1974. *Prevention and Treatment of Mental Illness in The Peoples Republic of China*. Ortho-Psychiatry, 44(4): 620-636.
92. Jew, C. C. and S. A. Brody. 1967. *Mental Illness among the Chinese: Hospitalization Rates Over the Past Century*. Psychiatry, 8(2): 129-134.
93. Kleinman, A. and T. Lin. 1981. *Normal and Abnormal Behavior in Chinese Culture*. Boston: D. Reidel Publishing Co.
94. Koran, L. M. 1972. *Psychiatry in Mainland China: History and Recent Status, Psychiatry*. 128(8): 970-977.

95. Lamson, H. D. 1935. *Social Pathology in China*. Shanghai: The Commercial Press.
96. Tseng, W. *The Development of Psychiatric Concepts and Traditional Chinese Medicine, Arch. Gen. Psychiatry*. 29: 569-575.
97. Zhi-zhong, Li. 1984. *Traditional Chinese Concepts of Mental Health*, AMA. 252(22): 31–69.

Chapter 7. A Comparison of the Five Cultures

A. The discussion of child abuse in society utilized many clinical experiences and references. Of particularly great help were the following, which contain general and specific points that I drew upon to compile the list in the text:

Breiner, S. J. 1979. *Psychological Factors in Violent Persons*, Psychological Reports, 44: 91-103.

Erikson, E. 1950. *Childhood and Society*, New York: W. W. Norton.

Finkelhor, D. 1984. *Child Sexual Abuse*, New York: The Free Press.

Herbolsheimer, H. 1985. AMA Diagnostic and Treatment Guidelines on Child Abuse and Neglect, *Report of the Council on Scientific Affairs of the AMA*, JAMA, 254(6) 796-800.

Humphrey, J. P. and H. J. Kupferer, 1977. *Pockets of Violence: An Exploration of Homicide and Suicide*, DNS, 38: 833-837.

National Opinion Research Center, University of Chicago, Brandeis University, Oct. 1965.

Pelton, L. H., ed. 1985. *The Social Context of Child Abuse and Neglect*. New York: Sciences Press.

Porterfield, A. L. and R. H. Filbert, 1948. *Crime, Suicide and Social Well Being*. Ft. Worth, Texas: Leo Potisham Foundation.

Schlosser, P. T. 1964. *The Abused Child, Bull. Menninger Clinic*, 28.

Simmons, B., E. Downs, M. Horster, and M. Archer. 1966. *Child Abuse Survey*. New York: Columbia University School of Public Health.

Strauss, M. and J. Strauss. 1953. *Suicide, Homicide and Social Structure in Ceylon, AJ of Sociology*, 58: 461-469.

B. The study of and writing about the family has been a particular interest of mine for years. But, to make the generalities that I compiled in the list "Child Abuse in the Family" more specific, especially for those who wish to explore the subject in greater depth, I have listed the following sources:

Ayoub, C. C. and J. S. Milner. 1985. *Failure to Thrive: Parental Indicators, Types, and Outcomes, Journal Child Abuse and Neglect.* Pergamon, 9: 4, 491-499.

Benedek, T. 1959. *Parenthood as a Development Phase*, JAPsychoanalytic Assoc. 7: 3, 389-417.

Berman, S. 1979. *The Psycho-Dynamic Aspects of Behavior*, Basic Handbook of Child Psychiatry, ed. J. P. Noshpitz. New York: Basic Books. 2.

Breiner, S. J. 1979. Psychological Factors in Violent Persons, *Psychological Reports,* 44: 91-103.

Cath, S. and C. Cath. 1978. *On the Other Side of Oz: Psychoanalytic Study of the Child.* New Haven, Conn.: Yale University Press.

Conte, J. R. and D. A. Shore, eds. 1982. *Social Work and Child Sexual Abuse, J. Soc. Work Hum. Sexuality.* New York: Haworth Press.

Davis, C. A. and D. Graybill. 1983. Comparison of the Family Environments of Abused Versus Non-Abused Children, *Psychology*, 20:1, 34-37.

Elmer, E. 1977. A Follow Up Study of Traumatized Children, *J. Ped.* 59: 273-279.

Erikson, E. 1950. *Childhood.* New York: W. W. Norton.

Finkelhor, D. 1984. *Child Sexual Abuse.* New York: The Free Press.

Fischhoff, J. *Failure to Thrive*, Basic Handbook of Child Psychiatry, J. Noshpitz, ed. New York: Basic Books, IV: 113-120.

Galdston, R. 1981. The Domestic Dimensions of Violence, *Psychoanalytic Study of the Child*, 36: 391-414.

Galdston, R. 1979. Disorders of Early Parenthood, *Basic Handbook of Child Psychiatry.* J. P. Noshpitz, ed. New York: Basic Books. 2: 581-593.

Groth, N. A. and J. Birnbaum, 1978. Adult Sexual Orientation and the Attraction to Underage Persons, *Arch. Sexual Behavior*, 7: 175-181.

Groth, N. A., W. Horace, and T. Gary, 1982. *The Child Molester: Clinical Observations*, in J. Conte and D. Shore, eds. *Social Work & Child Sexual Abuse.* New York: Haworth.

Groth, N. A. and A. W. Burgess, 1979. Sexual Trauma in the Life Histories of Rapists and Child Molesters, *Victimology*, 4: 10-16.

Halleck, S. L. 1976. Psychodynamic Aspects Of Violence, *Bull. Am. Acad. Psychiatry and Law*, 4: 328-335.

Harrison, S. and J. McDermott, Jr. 1980. *New Directions in Childhood Psychopathology*, New York: International Universities Press.

Helfer, R., E. Kemp, and C. Henry. 1968. *The Battered Child.* Chicago, Ill.: University of Chicago Press.

Kaufman, I. 1962. *Psychiatric Implications of Physical Abuse of Children,* Protecting the Battered Child. Children's Division, American Humane Assoc., Denver, Colo.

Marmor, J. ed. 1980. *Homosexual Behavior.* New York: Basic Books.

Merrill, E. J. 1962. *Protecting the Battered Child.* The American Humane Assoc., Denver, Colo.

Moll, A. 1913. *The Sexual Life of the Child.* New York: Macmillan and Co.

Morris, M. G. and R. W. Gould 1963. *The Neglected-Battered Child Syndrome.* Child Welfare League of America, New York.

National Opinion Research Center. 1965. University of Chicago and Brandeis University, Oct.

Panton, J. H. 1978. *Personality Differences Appearing Between Rapists of Adults, Rapists of Children and Non-Violent Sexual Molesters of Children,* Research Communications in Psychology, Psychiatry and Behavior, 3(4): 385-393.

Pasternak, E. ed. *Violence and Victims.* New York: Spectrum.

Pelton, L. H. ed. 1985. *The Social Context of Child Abuse and Neglect.* New York: Human Sciences Press.

Russell, D. 1984. *Sexual Exploitation: Rape, Child Sexual Abuse, and Sexual Harassment.* Beverly Hills, Calif.: Sage.

Sadoff, R. L. 1971. *Clinical Observations on Parricide, Psychiatric Quarterly.* 45: 65-69.

Sargent, D. 1971. *The Lethal Situation: Transmission of Urge to Kill from Parent to Child,* In J. Fawcett, ed. *Dynamics of Violence.* Chicago: AMA, 105-113.

Schlosser, P. T. 1964. *The Abused Child,* Menninger Clinic, 28, Sept.

Simmons, B., E. Downs, M. Horster, and M. Archer, 1966. *Child Abuse.*

Steele, B. F. and C. B. Pollock, 1968. A Psychiatric Study of Parents Who Abuse Infants and Small Children, *The Battered Child,* Helfer and Kempe, eds. Chicago, Ill: University of Chicago Press.

Swanson, D. W. 1968. *Adult Sexual Abuse of Children: The Man and Circumstances, Dis. Nerv. Sys.,* 29: 677-683.

Chapter 8. The Psychodynamics of Child Abuse

A. This list is a composite of individual characteristics gathered from the following references:

Berman, S. 1979. *The Psycho-Dynamic Aspects of Behavior*, in *Basic Handbook of Child Psychiatry*, Vol. 2, J. P. Noshpitz, ed. New York: Basic Books.

Breiner, S. J. 1979. Psychological Factors in Violent Persons, *Psychological Reports*, 44: 91-103.

Cath, S. and C. Cath, 1978. On the Other Side of Oz, *Psychoanalytic Study of the Child*, New Haven, Conn.: Yale University Press. 33.

Finkelhor, D. 1984. *Child.*

Galdston, R. 1981. The Domestic Dimensions of Violence, *Psychoanalytic Study of the Child*, 36: 391-414.

Galdston, R. 1979. *Disorders.*

Groth, N. A. and A. W. Burgess. 1979. *Sexual Trauma.*

Halleck, S. L. 1976. *Psychodynamic.*

Harrison, S. and J. McDermott, Jr. 1980. *New Directions.*

Helfer, R., E. Kemp, and C. Henry. 1968. *The Battered.*

Kaufman, I. 1982. *Psychiatric Implications.*

Merrill, E. J. 1962. *Protecting.*

Morris, M. G. and R. W. Gould. 1963. *The Neglected-Battered Child Syndrome*. New York: Child Welfare League of America.

Panton, J. 1979. MMPI Profile Configurations Associated with Incestuous and Non-Incestuous Child Molesting. *Psychological Reports*, 45: 335-338.

Panton, J. H. 1978. *Personality Differences.*

Pasternak, E. ed. 1975. *Violence and Victims*, New York: Spectrum.

Steele, B. F. and C. B. Pollock. 1968. *A Psychiatric Study.*

Zetzel, E. R. 1953. *The Oppressive Position, Affective Disorders*, P. Greenacre, ed. New York: International Universities Press.

B. This section on our society has more specific references; however, some general observations about our society related to child abuse are based on material from these references:

Davis, C. A. and D. Graybill. 1983. *Comparison.*

Fillippi, R. K. 1979. *Child Abuse*, in *Basic Handbook of Child Psychiatry*, J. P. Noshpitz, ed. Basic Books, 4: 364-374.

Humphrey, J. P. and H. J. Kupferer. 1977. *Pockets.*

Simmons, B., E. Downs, M. Horster, and M. Archer, *Child Abuse.*

C. The topic of sexual abuse has an extensive literature, from which many references are specifically cited in the text. In addition I have listed the following since I have utilized their information in formulating many of my ideas:

Conte, J. R. and D. A. Shore, eds. 1982. *Social Work.*
Finkelhor, D. 1984. *Child.*
Groth, N. and J. Birnbaum. 1978. *Adult.*
Groth, N. A., W. Horace, and T. Gary. 1982. *The Child Molester.*
Groth, N. A. and A. W. Burgess. 1979. *Sexual Trauma.*
Marmor, J., ed. 1980. *Homosexual.*
Moll, A. 1913. *The Sexual Life.*
Panton, J. H. 1978. *Personality.*
Russell, D. 1984. *Sexual Exploitation.*
Swanson, D. W. 1968. *Adult.*

1. Hausfactor, G. and S. B. Hrdy. 1984. *Infanticide.*
2. Berman, S. 1979. *The Psycho-Dynamic.*
3. Breiner, S. J. 1979. *Psychological Factors.*
4. Spitz, R. 1958. On the Genesis of Superego Components, in *Psychoanalytic Study of The Child,* 13.
5. Helfer, R., E. Kemp, and C. Henry. 1968. *The Battered.*
6. Pasternak, E., ed. 1975. *Violence.*
7. Breiner, S. J. 1979. *Psychological Factors.*
8. Pasternak, E. ed. 1979. *Violence.*
9. Dunn, C. 1920. *The National History of the Child.* New York: John Layne, Publishers.
10. Erikson, E. 1950. *Childhood.*
11. Moll, A. 1913. *The Sexual.*
12. Spitz, R. 1958. *On The Genesis.*
13. Breiner, S. J. 1979. *Psychological Factors.*
14. Ibid.
15. Conte, J. R. and D. A. Shore, eds. 1982. *Social Work.*
16. Galdston, R. 1981. *The Domestic.*
17. Hausfactor, G. and S. B. Hrdy. 1984. *Infanticide.*
18. Helfer, R., E. Kemp, and C. Henry. 1968. *The Battered.*
19. Pasternak, E. ed. 1975. *Violence.*
20. Strauss, M. and J. Strauss. 1953. *Suicide, Homicide and Social Structure in Ceylon, A. J. Sociol.* 58: 461-469.
21. Porterfield, A. L. and R. H. Filbert. 1948. *Crime.*
22. Herbolsheimer, H. 1985. *AMA Diagnostic.*
23. Halleck, S. L. 1976. *Psychodynamic.*

24. Sadoff, R. L. 1971. Clinical Observations on Parricide, *Psychiatric Quarterly*, 45: 65-69.
25. Sargent, D. 1971. *The Lethal.*
26. Breiner, S. J. 1979. *Psychological Factors.*
27. Pasternak, E., ed. 1975. *Violence.*
28. Breiner, S. J. 1979. *Psychological Factors.*
29. Harrison, S. and J. McDermott, Jr. 1980. *New Directions.*
30. Pelton, L. H., ed. 1985. *The Social Context.*
31. Schlosser, P. T. 1964. *The Abused.*
32. Simmons, B. *et al.* 1966. *Child Abuse.*
33. National Opinion. 1965.
34. Ibid.
35. Benedek, T. 1959. *Parenthood.*
36. Breiner, S. J. 1979. *Psychological Factors.*
37. Davis, C. A. and D. Graybill. 1983. *Comparison.*
38. Galdston, R. 1979. *Disorders.*
39. Steele, B. F. and C. B. Pollock, 1968. *A Psychiatric Study.*
40. Cath, S. and C. Cath. 1978. On the Other Side of Oz, *Psychoanalytic Study of the Child.* New Haven, Conn.: Yale University Press.
41. Kaufman, I. 1962. *Psychiatric Implications.*
42. Steele, B. F. and C. B. Pollock. 1968. *A Psychiatric Study.*
43. Morris, M. G. and R. W. Gould. 1963. *The Neglected.*
44. Conte, J. R. and D. A. Shore, eds. 1982. *Social Work.*
45. Fillippi, R. K. 1979. *Child.*
46. Helfer, R., E. Kemp, and C. Henry. 1968. *The Battered Child.*
47. Morris, M. G. and R. W. Gould. 1963. *The Neglected.*
48. Pelton, L. H., ed. 1985. *The Social Context.*
49. Schlosser, P. T. 1964. *The Abused.*
50. Steele, B. F. and C. B. Pollock. 1968. *A Psychiatric Study.*
51. Merrill and Heins. 1984. *The Battered Child Revisited*, JAMA, 251.24: 3295-3300.
52. Davis, C. A. and D. Graybill. 1983. *Comparison.*
53. Elmer, E. 1977. *A Follow-Up.*
54. Helfer, R., E. Kemp, and C. Henry. 1968. *The Battered.*
55. Ibid.
56. Steele, B. F. and C. B. Pollock. 1968. *A Psychiatric Study.*
57. Galdston, R. 1981. *The Domestic Dimensions.*
59. Steele, B. F. and C. B. Pollock. 1968. *A Psychiatric Study.*
60. Erikson, E. 1950. *Childhood.*
61. Fischhoff, J. 1979. *Failure to Thrive.*
62. Russell, D. 1984. *Sexual Exploitation.*

63. Finkelhor, D. 1984. *Child.*
64. Groth, N. and J. Birnbaum. 1978. *Adult.*
65. Groth, N. and A. Burgess. *Motivational Intent.*
66. Groth, N. A., W. Horace, and T. Gary. 1982. *The Child Molester.*
67. Groth, N. A. and A. W. Burgess. 1979. *Sexual Trauma.*
68. Panton, J. H. 1978. *Personality.*
69. Swanson, D. W. 1968. *Adult.*
70. Panton, J. 1979. *MMPI Profile.*
71. Panton, J. H. 1978. *Personality.*
72. Finkelhor, D. 1984. *Child.*
73. Russell, D. 1980. *The Prevalence and Impact of Marital Rape in San Francisco.* Paper presented to the American Sociological Association, New York.
74. Russell, D. 1984. *Sexual Exploitation.*
75. Conte, J. R. and D. A. Shore, eds. 1982. *Social Work.*
76. Finkelhor, D. 1984. *Child.*
77. Groth, N. A. and A. W. Burgess. 1979.
78. Finkelhor, D. 1984. *Child.*
79. Ibid.
80. Ibid.
81. Russell, D. 1984. *Sexual Exploitation.*
82. Galdston, R. 1981. *The Domestic Dimensions.*
83. Galdston, R. 1979. *Disorders.*
84. Galdston, R. 1981. *The Domestic Dimensions.*
85. Galdston, R. 1979. *Disorders.*
86. Humphrey, J. P. and H. J. Kupferer. 1977. *Pockets.*

Chapter 9. Conclusion: Our Future from the Past

1. Hausfactor, G. and S. B. Hrdy, eds. 1984. *Infanticide.*
2. Galdston, R. 1981. *The Domestic.*
3. Davis, C. A. and D. Graybill. 1983. *Comparison.*
4. Erikson, E. 1950. *Childhood.*
5. Sargent, D. 1971. *The Lethal Situation.*
6. Menninger, K. 1954. Psychological Aspects of the Organism Under Stress: Part I The Homeostatic Regulatory Function of the Ego, *J. A. Psychoanalytic Assoc.* 2: 67-106.
7. Breiner, S. J. 1979. *Psychological Factors.*
8. Davis, C. A. and D. Graybill. 1983. *Comparison.*
9. Benedek, T. 1959. *Parenthood.*

10. Erikson, E. 1950. *Childhood*.
11. Cath, S. and C. Cath. 1978. *On the Other Side*.
12. Kaufman, I. 1962. *Psychiatric Implications*.
13. Steele, B. F. and C. B. Pollock. 1968. *A Psychiatric Study*.
14. Ibid.
15. Merrill, E. J. 1962. *Protecting*.
16. Davis, C. A. and D. Graybill. 1983. *Comparison*.
17. Galdston, R. 1981. *The Domestic Dimensions*.
18. Galdston, R. 1979. *Disorders*.
19. Kaufman, I. 1962. *Psychiatric Implications*.
20. Morris, M. G. and R. W. Gould. 1963. *The Neglected*.
21. Schlosser, P. T. 1964. *The Abused*.
22. Steele, B. F. and C. B. Pollock. 1968. *A Psychiatric Study*.
23. Ibid.
24. Pelton, L. H. ed. 1985. *The Social Context*.
25. Benedek, T. 1959. *Parenthood*.
26. Bettelheim, B. 1969. *The Children of the Dream*. New York: Macmillan.

Index

Children (*Cont.*)
  as human sacrifice
    in China, 142
    in Crete, 37-38
    in Greece, 37-38, 43, 49
    by Hebrews, 67, 68, 249
    in Rome, 117-118
  identification with parents, 246
  illegitimacy/legitimacy, 19, 44-45,
    50, 78
  motherless, 179
  murder by, 211
  murder of
    Germanic tribes' prohibition of,
      119
    of grown children, 183
    by parents, 107, 221-222
    in Rome, 117, 118
    See also Infanticide
  as oracles, 17
  punishment, 88, 178, 247
    corporal punishment, 79, 113,
      190, 220, 240, 248, 262
  religious concepts of, 253
  rights, 258, 259
  sale of, 79, 80, 96, 119
  as slaves, 171, 172, 237-238, 250
  starvation, 112
  suicide, 210
  torture, 120
  walking age, 115
China, 129-185, 197-198
  ancestor worship, 133, 140-142,
    153, 160
  architecture, 138
  capital punishment, 137
  childrearing practices, 147-148,
    172-178, 179
  children, 147-148, 250, 251, 254
    passivity, 177
    punishment, 178
  Chin dynasty, 133
  Ching dynasty, 159, 165, 250
  Chou dynasty, 131, 143, 163
  cultural characteristics, 192

China (*Cont.*)
  education, 147-148, 176, 177-178
  family, 140-141, 189, 255
    government standards for,
      149-150
  fathers, 149, 159, 175, 183, 252
    relations with son, 141, 144-145,
      146-147, 155, 255, 256
  geography, 130-131
  Han dynasty, 133, 136, 165, 166,
    167, 171-173, 183
  history of civilization, 129-143
  homosexuality, 157, 164-165, 166
  human sacrifice, 133, 142, 171, 197
  infanticide, 144, 146, 156, 178,
    179-181, 182, 183, 192, 197, 250
  inheritance, 145, 147, 158, 182
  legal system, 151-157, 198
  Manchu dynasty, 138-139, 169
  marriage, 145-146, 158, 162-163,
    176, 198
  matriarchy, 162
  medical care, 182
  mentally ill, 183-185, 197
  Ming dynasty, 137, 150, 167, 168,
    170, 182, 250
  Mongol dynasty, 138, 150, 159,
    161, 168, 170, 181, 182, 250
  religion, 140, 197-198. *See also*
    China, ancestor worship
  remarriage, 146
  sexual attitudes, 161-167
  Shun dynasty, 131
  slavery, 133, 136-137, 155, 170-172,
    178, 197
  social classes, 144
  Sui dynasty, 134
  Sung dynasty, 137
  Tang dynasty, 137, 163, 167, 180,
    183
  torture, 143, 156-157
  women, 140, 145, 146, 150-160,
    198, 251
    Confucian view of, 165
    as criminals, 151, 152, 153, 157

China (*Cont.*)
  women (*Cont.*)
    footbinding, 168-170
    legal rights, 155
    magical powers, 161
    religious duties, 142
    sexual freedom, 157
    sexual knowledge, 161-162, 163,
      166-167
    sexual rights, 165-166
    suicide, 183
  xenophobia, 139
  Yao dynasty, 131
  Yin dynasty, 131
  Yuan dynasty, 182
Chin dynasty, 133
Chinese-Americans, 184-185, 216
Ching dynasty, 159, 165, 250
Ch'in Shih-huang, 152
Chou Code, 151
Chou dynasty, 131, 143, 163
Christianity
  in China, 140
  marital relationship in, 74
Christians, belief in pagan gods, 103
Cicero, 103
Circumcision
  in Egypt, 21, 75
  in Greece, 42
  of Hebrews, 75, 95
  of Mohammedans, 75
City-states
  Greek, 38-39, 40, 58
  Roman, 108-109
Civil service system
  of China, 148
  of Egypt, 22
  of Rome, 126
Clairvoyancy, 102
Clock, invention, 28
Code of Hammurabi, 94
Code of the Hittites, 94
Coitus interruptus, 116
Colosseum, 99-100
Commodus, 126

Concubinage
  in Greece, 44-45, 47
  homosexual, 49
  among Hebrews, 95, 96
  in Rome, 113
Concubines
  children of, 44-45
  in China, 158, 167, 168
    of king, 160, 161
    sexual rights, 166
  living burial, 160
  of pharaohs, 23
Confucianism, 140, 152, 157, 163
Confucius, 135-136, 145, 171
  view of women, 165
Conscience, 208-209
Constantine, Emperor, 102, 115
Constantinople, 102
Constitution, first, 68
Contraception
  birth control planning, 257
  Hebrews' use of, 82-83
  Romans' use of, 116, 117
Corporal punishment
  child abuse correlation, 190, 220,
    248
  child abuse versus, 240
  of Hebrew children, 79
  legal prohibition, 262
  of Roman children, 113
Corsica, 101
Courtesans
  in China, 167-168
  in Greece, 41, 42
Cousins, marriage of, 145-146
Covenant of Abraham, 42
Crete
  destruction, 38
  Egyptian influences on, 37
  Etruscans' relationship with, 100
  pre-Mycenae, 37
  women's status, 43
Criminals
  in China, 151, 152, 153, 157
  in Egypt, 26, 27

Mother (*Cont.*)
  depression of, 252
  of "failure to thrive" children,
    224-225
  infanticide by, 203
  of sexually-abused children,
    227-228, 230, 231
Mother–child relationship
  as child abuse factor, 246, 254
  in China, 141, 172
  in Egypt, 14-15
  in "failure to thrive," 224-225
  psychological factors, 20
  separation effects, 255
Mother Goddess, 43
Motherhood, preparation for,
    260-261, 262-263
Mount Sinai, 69
Mourning practices
  Chinese, 141, 198
  Hebrew, 195
Mummification, 30
Murder
  of children
    Germanic tribes' prohibition of,
      119
    of grown children, 183
    by parents, 107, 221-222
    in Rome, 117, 118
    by Egyptian gods, 25
    Hebrew law regarding, 86, 86
    by Judean kings, 68
    by minors, 211
    as self-aggression, 210
    of slaves, 122, 123
Murderer, cities of refuge for, 88-89
Musonius Rufus, 113
Mutilation
  of children, 111
  of slaves, 123
Mycenae, 37-38, 39, 43

Necco II, Pharaoh, 30
Nepal, child slavery, 238
Nero, Emperor, 110, 119-120, 122

Newborn, Egyptian attitudes toward,
    17
Niddah, 84
Nietzsche, Friedrich, 62
Nightmares, 115
Noah, 69
Nubia, 14, 26
Nudity, 25, 193
Nut (goddess), 30

Octavian, Emperor, 101
Oedipal complex, 205-206
Oikos, 40, 45-46
Old Testament, 65
Olympic games, 42, 59
Olympus, 57
Omophagia, 41
On, King, 65-66
Onanism, 79
Oracle, children as, 17
Orgies, Roman, 120
Orphans
  in Egypt, 17-19
  Hebrew law regarding, 87
Osiris, 17, 29
Ostrogoths, 102

Pakistan, child slavery, 238
Palestine, 64, 67
Parent
  child-abusing
    characteristics, 217-221, 222,
      239-248
    childhood abuse of, 244-245
    mother–child relationship, 245,
      246
    parental relations, 253-254
    psychosis of, 241-242
  of "failure to thrive" children,
    223-225
  murder of children by, 107,
    221-222
Parthia, 134
Pater familias, 105-106, 145

Prostitution (*Cont.*)
  in Rome, 111, 117, 118
Psychosis
  of child-abusing parents, 241-242
  ego functioning and, 210, 243
Psychotherapy, for child abuse prevention, 257-258
Ptah-hotep, Pharaoh, 31
Ptolemaic pharaohs, 28, 39, 188, 249, 252
Ptolemy, 39
Pubic hair, depilation, 42
Public schools, Hebrew, 90
Punic Wars, 101
Punishment
  of children, 88, 178, 247
  See also Corporal punishment
Pyramids, 30
Pyrrhus, 58
Pythagoras, School of, 47

Queen, sexual activity of, 160-161
Quintilian, 113, 114

Racial factors, in child abuse, 213, 214-215, 218
Rain god/goddess, 143, 162
Ramses II, Pharaoh, 21, 67, 249
Ramses III, Pharaoh, 33
Rape
  in China, 156
  in Greece, 43
  Hebrew concept of, 83, 86
  homosexual, 122, 157
  in Rome, 114
Re, 29, 30
Reality
  child's perception of, 209
  detachment from, 241, 243
Rebecca, 84
Reincarnation, 141
Religion
  of Chinese, 140, 197-198
  of Egyptians, 29-30, 188, 192

Religion (*Cont.*)
  of Hebrews, 64-65, 66, 68, 69-70, 74, 76-77, 78, 85-86, 92, 93-94, 97
  of Romans, 102-105
  See also God(s); Goddesses
Religious factors, in child abuse, 253
Remarriage, 111, 146
Rhea, 57
Ricci, Matteo, 182
River god, 142-143
Roman Way, The (Hamilton), 106
Rome, 99-128, 196-197
  adoption, 106
  adultery, 106
  barbarian invasions, 101-120
  child abuse, 112-115, 192, 196, 253
  childlessness, 116
  children, 105, 106, 188, 249-250, 251, 252
    murder of, 117
  city-states, 108-109
  civil service, 126
  civil war, 109
  conquest of Greece, 111
  cultural characteristics, 192
  division of, 102
  education, 112, 196-197
  fall of, 136
  family, 109, 251
  father–son relationship, 104-105
  Greek influences on, 101, 112
  homosexuality, 111, 113, 114, 126
  infanticide, 107, 111, 116, 117, 118, 126
  inheritance, 105, 116
  legal system, 106-107, 117, 123-124, 125-127, 197, 250
  marriage, 116, 126, 196
  marriage age, 110
  mercenaries, 111
  origins, 100, 101
  pater familias, 105-106, 145
  population decline, 111
  population growth, 108